# A Handy
# Sodium Diet
# Cookbook

Easy & Delicious Low Sodium Recipes

BY: SOPHIA FREEMAN

HOME
FOOD
The best recipe

# Table of Contents

# Introduction

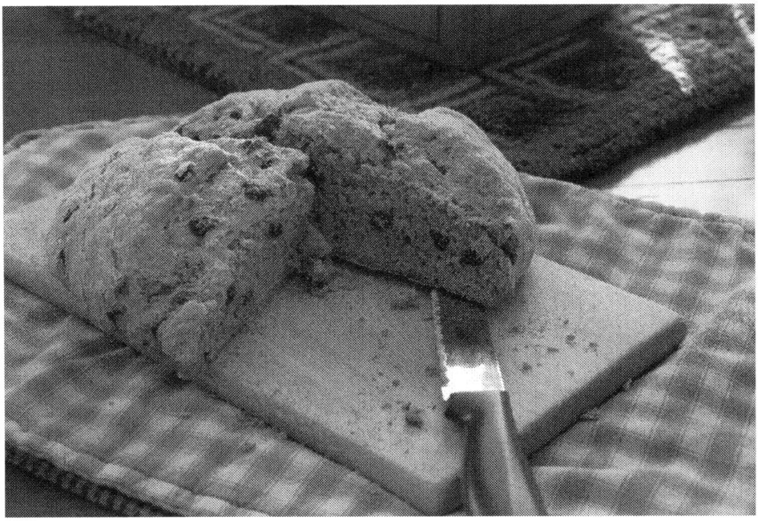

Some foods naturally contain sodium.

Its most common form is sodium chloride, more popularly known as the table salt.

Sodium is also added in some food products.

Fast food items and instant food products are known for containing high amounts of sodium.

People need a minimum of 500 milligrams of sodium a day.

But some consume 3,000 milligrams or more daily.

This can pose serious negative effects on one's health. High sodium has been linked to numerous health problems including but not limited to heart disease, kidney stones, kidney failure and hypertension.

It is therefore important to maintain a low sodium diet in which consumption ranges only between 1,500 and 2,400 milligrams per day.

In this cookbook, you will find 50 low-sodium recipes, all of which are made with healthy and natural ingredients and will not take too much of your time and effort.

Some recipes indicate long hours of cooking but take note that the active preparation time is usually only a few minutes.

Make sure too that when you encounter the "salt to taste" ingredient in the recipe, you only use a small pinch, ideally 1/8 teaspoon.

Here's to a start of a healthier diet and lifestyle for you.

# Braised Beef with Dried Apricots & Cranberries

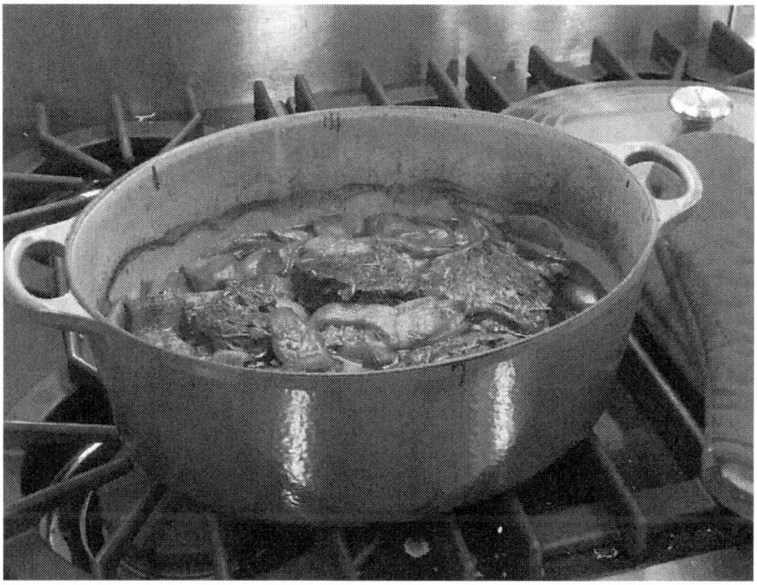

Brisket is tougher than other cuts of beef, which is why it is often braised in sauce or slow cooked to make it tender. In this recipe, we'll be braising beef brisket and adding dried fruits like cranberries and apricots to create a tasty dish that you will absolutely love.

**Serving size:** 10

**Preparation Cooking Time:** 4 hours and 50 minutes

**Ingredients:**

- 3 star anise
- 1 teaspoon ground cinnamon
- 4 teaspoons cocoa powder (unsweetened)
- 2 teaspoons red pepper flakes, crushed
- 4 teaspoons ground sumac
- 4 lb. beef brisket, trimmed and sliced
- Salt to taste
- 2 tablespoons olive oil
- 8 cloves garlic, crushed and minced
- 4 white onions, sliced
- ¼ cup dried cranberries
- ¼ cup dried apricots
- ¼ cup raisins
- ¼ cup prunes, pitted
- 4 cups reduced-sodium beef broth
- 1 orange, sliced into wedges

**Instructions:**

1. Preheat your oven to 325 degrees F.

2. Add the star anise to a spice grinder.

3. Grind into powder.

4. Put the anise powder in a bowl.

5. Stir in the cinnamon, cocoa, red pepper flakes and ground sumac.

6. Sprinkle the beef with salt and half of the anise mixture.

7. Pour the oil into a pan over medium heat.

8. Cook the beef for 4 to 5 minutes per side.

9. Transfer to a plate.

10. Add the onions and cook for 10 minutes, stirring frequently.

11. Stir in the rest of the ingredients along with the remaining spice blend.

12. Bring to a boil and then simmer for 15 minutes.

13. Transfer the pan to the oven and bake for 3 hours and 30 minutes.

14. Pour the sauce over the beef and serve.

**Nutrients per Serving:**

- Calories 290
- Fat 9 g
- Saturated fat 3 g
- Carbohydrates 16 g
- Fiber 2 g
- Protein 36 g
- Cholesterol 98 mg
- Sugars 10 g
- Sodium 320 mg
- Potassium 758 mg

# Stir-fried Tofu Mushrooms

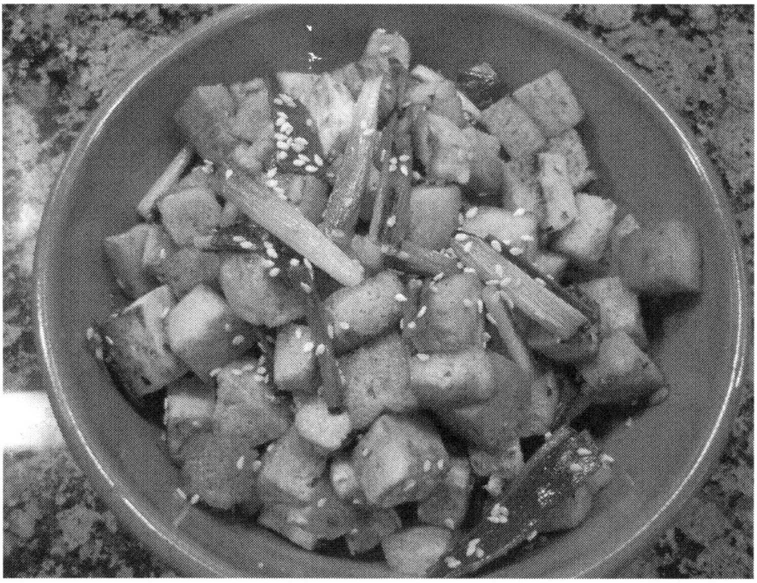

Looking for a quick meal to prepare during a busy weeknight? Here's one that will only take you less than an hour to prepare. You'll love the crunchy tofu flavored with sesame and teriyaki sauce.

**Serving size:** 5

**Preparation Cooking Time:** 20 minutes

**Ingredients:**

- 4 tablespoons vegetable oil, divided
- 1 red bell pepper, diced
- ½ lb. mushroom buttons
- ½ lb. shiitake mushrooms
- 1 clove garlic, grated
- 1 tablespoon fresh ginger, grated
- 2 stalks scallions, sliced
- 8 oz. tofu, baked crispy
- 3 teaspoons reduced-sodium oyster sauce

**Instructions:**

1. Pour half the oil into a pan over medium high heat.

2. Cook and stir the bell pepper and mushrooms for 4 minutes.

3. Add the garlic, ginger and scallions.

4. Cook for 30 seconds, stirring frequently.

5. Transfer the bell pepper mixture into a bowl.

6. Pour in the remaining oil.

7. Cook the tofu for 4 minutes.

8. Put your vegetables back to the pan and season with the oyster sauce.

9. Cook while stirring for 1 to 2 minutes.

**Nutrients per Serving:**

- Calories 171
- Fat 13 g
- Saturated fat 2 g
- Carbohydrates 9 g
- Fiber 2 g
- Protein 8 g
- Cholesterol 0 mg
- Sugars 3 g
- Sodium 309 mg
- Potassium 469 mg

# Baked White Fish with Quinoa Veggies

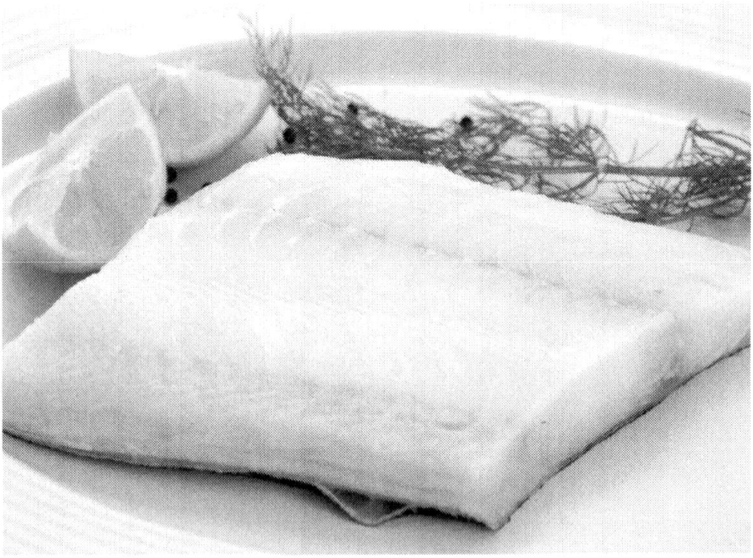

One look at this dish and you might want to skip it because it looks complicated. Not only do you have to cook the fish, you also have to prepare two sides. But you'll be surprised when you find out that all these come together in less than an hour.

**Serving size:** 4

**Preparation Cooking Time:** 30 minutes

**Ingredients:**

- 1 bulb fennel, sliced into strips
- 1 lb. Brussels sprouts, sliced in half
- 2 tablespoons olive oil, divided
- Salt and pepper to taste
- 4 white fish fillets
- 4 cloves garlic, crushed, minced and divided
- 2 tablespoons butter (unsalted)
- 3 tablespoons freshly squeezed lemon juice
- 2 cups quinoa, cooked
- ¼ cup sun-dried tomatoes, sliced
- 2 tablespoons parsley, chopped
- ¼ cup Kalamata olives, pitted and chopped

**Instructions:**

1. Preheat your oven to 400 degrees F.

2. Toss the fennel strips and Brussels sprouts in 1 teaspoon olive oil and season with the salt and pepper.

3. Arrange in a baking pan.

4. Bake for 20 minutes.

5. While waiting, add the fish fillets to another baking pan, sprinkled with half of the garlic and seasoned with salt and pepper.

6. In a bowl, mix the butter and lemon juice with 1 tablespoon olive oil.

7. Brush both sides of the fish with this mixture.

8. Bake in the oven for 12 minutes.

9. Mix the quinoa, remaining oil, tomatoes, parsley and olives.

10. Serve the fish with the roasted veggies and quinoa mixture.

**Nutrients per Serving:**

- Calories 406
- Fat 17 g
- Saturated fat 5 g
- Carbohydrates 36 g
- Fiber 8 g
- Protein 30 g
- Cholesterol 71 mg
- Sugars 5 g
- Sodium 560 mg
- Potassium 1379 mg

# Fish Curry Stew

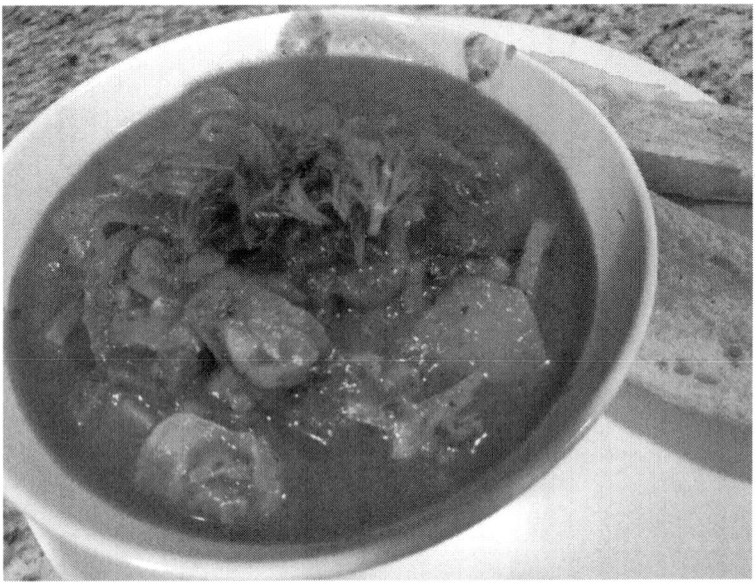

One thing that you'd love about this dish is how the sweet potatoes lend creamy rich flavor t to the stew, and the curry a bit of spice. It's a quick recipe that takes about 50 minutes or so to prepare.

**Serving size:** 4

**Preparation Cooking Time:** 45 minutes

**Ingredients:**

- 1 tablespoon vegetable oil
- 1 tablespoon garlic, chopped
- 1 tablespoon ginger, chopped
- 2 sweet potatoes, sliced into cubes
- 1 yellow bell pepper, sliced
- Salt to taste
- 1 tablespoon curry powder
- 15 oz. coconut milk
- 4 cod fillets
- 2 teaspoons freshly squeezed lime juice
- 3 tablespoons cilantro, chopped
- 4 cups brown rice, cooked

**Instructions:**

1. Pour the oil into a pan over medium heat.

2. Cook the garlic and ginger for 30 seconds.

3. Stir in the sweet potatoes and bell pepper.

4. Season with the salt and curry powder.

5. Cook for 2 minutes.

6. Pour in the coconut milk.

7. Cover the pan.

8. Simmer for 15 minutes.

9. Put the cod fillets on top of the sweet potatoes.

10. Cover and cook for 8 minutes.

11. Drizzle the lime juice and add the cilantro.

12. Serve the fish curry stew with brown rice.

**Nutrients per Serving:**

- Calories 382
- Fat 11 g
- Saturated fat 5 g
- Carbohydrates 49 g
- Fiber 5 g
- Protein 19 g
- Cholesterol 45 mg
- Sugars 8 g
- Sodium 413 mg
- Potassium 736 mg

# Green Beans with Bacon

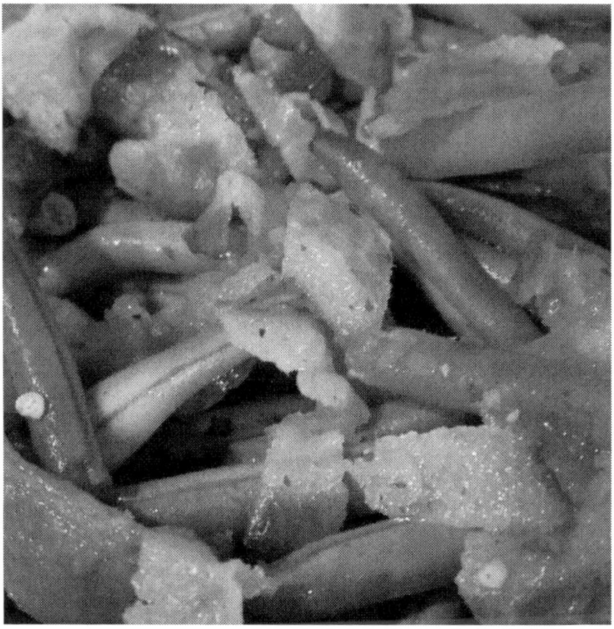

You might not have thought of this combination before, but these two actually go well together. Bacon adds extra flavor to the green beans, making these delicious veggies even more enticing.

**Serving size:** 8

**Preparation Cooking Time:** 30 minutes

**Ingredients:**

- 2 oz. bacon, chopped
- 24 oz. green beans, trimmed
- 1 stalk shallot, chopped
- Salt and pepper to taste
- ½ teaspoon smoked paprika
- 1 teaspoon freshly squeezed lemon juice
- 2 teaspoons red-wine vinegar

**Instructions:**

1. Preheat your oven to 450 degrees F.

2. Arrange the bacon slices on your baking pan.

3. Roast for 5 minutes.

4. Stir in the rest of the ingredients except the lemon juice and vinegar.

5. Roast for 12 minutes.

6. Add the lemon juice and vinegar in the last 2 minutes of cooking.

**Nutrients per Serving:**

- Calories 49
- Fat 1 g
- Saturated fat 0 g
- Carbohydrates 8 g
- Fiber 3 g
- Protein 3 g
- Cholesterol 3 mg
- Sugars 4 g
- Sodium 192 mg
- Potassium 249 mg

# Roasted Turkey

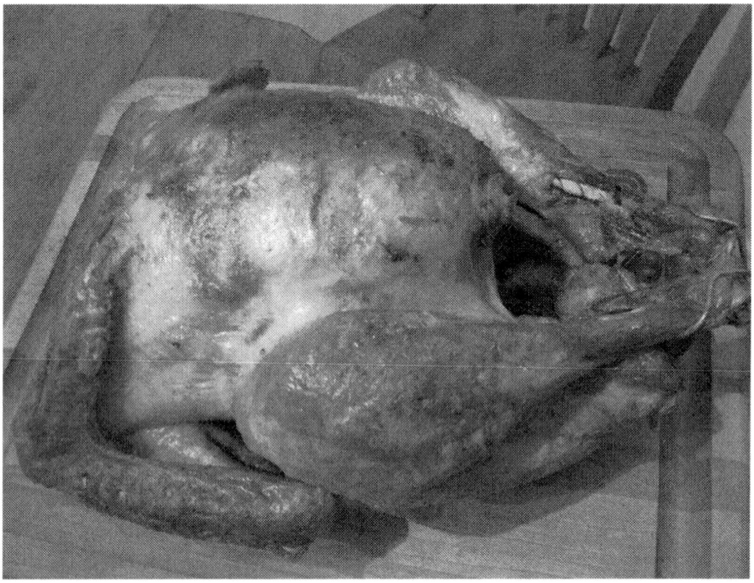

What makes this roasted turkey special? It's the herbed rub with garlic and lemon zest that gives this dish incredible flavor, plus the creamy gravy made from the pan drippings.

**Serving size:** 8

**Preparation Cooking Time:** 8 hours

**Ingredients:**

**Turkey:**

- 6 cloves garlic, crushed and minced
- 1 shallot, chopped
- 6 tablespoons butter (unsalted)
- 2 tablespoons rosemary, chopped
- 1½ teaspoons lemon zest
- 1½ tablespoons mustard

**Salt to taste:**

- 1 whole turkey, giblets and neck removed
- 1 onion, sliced into quarters
- 1 celery, sliced
- 1 carrot, sliced
- 1 lemon, sliced into half
- 5 sprigs thyme
- 5 sprigs rosemary
- 5 sprigs sage

**Gravy:**

- ¼ cup pan drippings from turkey
- 2 cloves garlic, crushed and minced
- 1 stalk shallot, minced
- ¼ cup all-purpose flour
- ½ cup dry white wine
- 3 cups reduced-sodium chicken broth
- 1 tablespoon sage, chopped
- 1 tablespoon thyme, chopped
- Salt and pepper to taste
- ¼ cup heavy cream

**Instructions:**

1. Mix the garlic, shallot, butter, rosemary, lemon zest, mustard and salt in a bowl.

2. Pat the turkey dry using paper towels.

3. Place the turkey on a baking pan.

4. Gently loosen the skin on all parts of the turkey.

5. Coat the whole turkey with the butter mixture including the meat underneath the skin.

6. Refrigerate the turkey for 4 hours.

7. Let sit in room temperature around 1 hour.

8. Preheat your oven to 450 degrees F.

9. Stuff the insides of the turkey with the remaining turkey ingredients.

10. Tuck the wings under and secure legs using kitchen string.

11. Roast in the oven for 30 minutes.

12. Reduce the temperature to 350 degrees F.

13. Roast for another 2 hours.

14. Transfer to a cutting board.

15. Take the pan drippings (1/4 cup) and set aside. Discard the rest of the drippings.

16. Transfer the drippings into a pan over medium heat.

17. Cook the garlic and shallot for 3 minutes.

18. Add the flour and cook for 2 minutes.

19. Stir in the wine and cook for 1 minute.

20. Stir in the rest of the ingredients except the cream and simmer for 12 minutes.

21. Strain the gravy.

22. Clean the pan. Put the gravy back to the pan and stir in the cream.

23. Cook on low heat for 5 minutes.

24. Slice the roasted turkey and serve with the gravy.

**Nutrients per Serving:**

- Calories 184
- Fat 7 g
- Saturated fat 3 g
- Carbohydrates 2 g
- Fiber 0 g
- Protein 26 g
- Cholesterol 79 mg
- Sugars 0 g
- Sodium 259 mg
- Potassium 233 mg

# Bell Peppers Stuffed with Quinoa, Chicken Parmesan

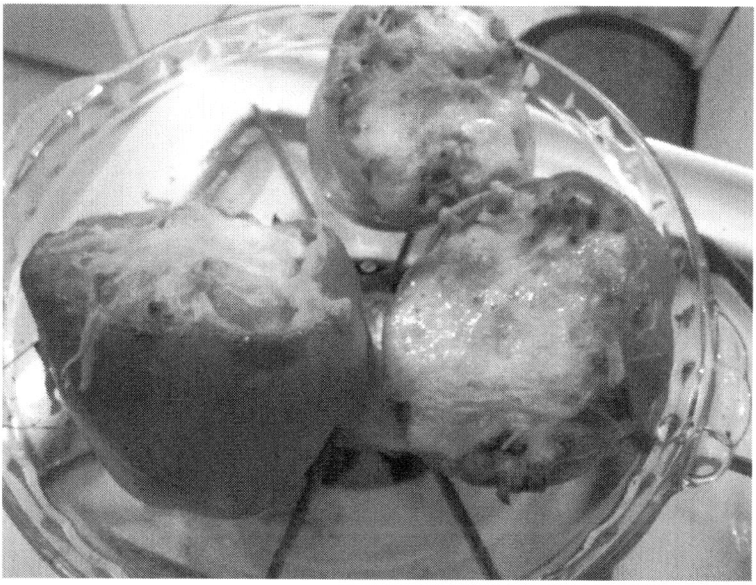

If you love chicken Parmesan, for sure, you'll also be delighted with this recipe in which the bell peppers are stuffed with chicken, Parmesan cheese, and quinoa.

**Serving size:** 4

**Preparation Cooking Time:** 1 hour

**Ingredients:**

- 1 tablespoon olive oil
- 2 cups onion, chopped
- 4 cloves garlic, crushed and minced
- 1 cup quinoa, rinsed and drained
- 1¼ cups water
- 2 cups reduced-sodium marinara sauce
- 3 cups chicken breast, cooked and shredded
- ½ cup Parmesan cheese, grated
- 1 cup fresh basil, chopped and divided
- 4 large bell peppers, tops trimmed
- ½ cup mozzarella cheese

**Instructions:**

1. Preheat your oven to 350 degrees F.

2. Pour the oil into a pan over medium heat.

3. Cook the onion and garlic for 5 minutes.

4. Stir in the quinoa and cook for 30 seconds.

5. Pour in the water.

6. Increase the heat to medium high and bring to a boil.

7. Slightly reduce the heat and simmer while covered for 15 minutes.

8. Remove from the stove.

9. Let sit for 5 minutes.

10. Add the marinara sauce, chicken, Parmesan cheese and half of the basil leaves.

11. Place the bell peppers on a baking pan.

12. Stuff each of the bell pepper with the chicken and quinoa mixture.

13. Roast in the oven for 15 minutes.

14. Sprinkle the top with the mozzarella cheese.

15. Roast for another 5 minutes.

16. Garnish with the remaining basil leaves.

**Nutrients per Serving:**

- Calories 559
- Fat 18 g
- Saturated fat 5 g
- Carbohydrates 49 g
- Fiber 8 g
- Protein 48 g
- Cholesterol 104 mg
- Sugars 13 g
- Sodium 522 mg
- Potassium 969 mg

# Maple Glazed Salmon

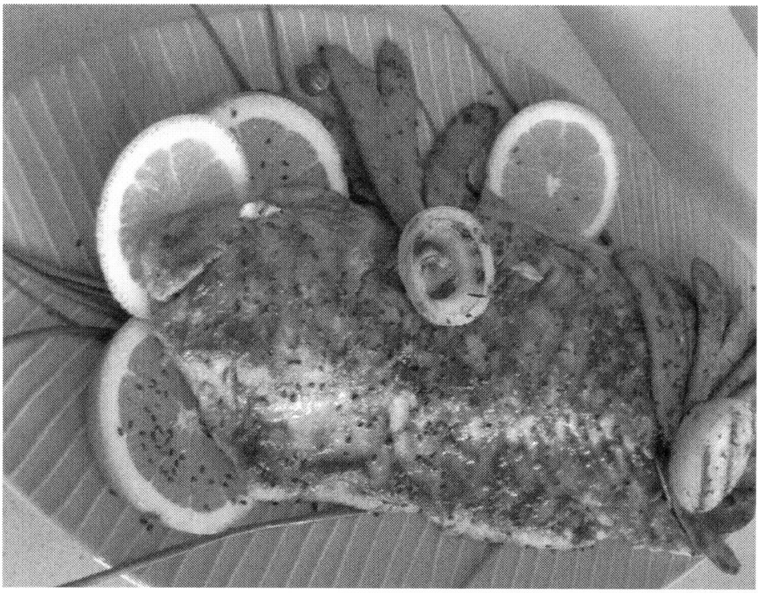

Among the many ways to cook salmon, this one is something that would forever stick in your memory because it packs in so much flavor and healthy goodness.

**Serving size:** 4

**Preparation Cooking Time:** 15 minutes

**Ingredients:**

- 1 tablespoon olive oil
- 1/8 cup white miso
- 1 tablespoon lemon juice
- 1 tablespoon lime juice
- Pepper to taste
- Pinch cayenne pepper
- 1 tablespoon maple syrup
- 4 salmon fillets
- Lemon slices

**Instructions:**

1. Cover your baking pan with foil.

2. In a bowl, mix the oil, miso, lemon juice, lime juice, cayenne, pepper, and maple syrup.

3. Brush both sides of the salmon with the miso mixture.

4. Place on the baking pan.

5. Top with the lemon slices.

6. Broil for 12 minutes.

**Nutrients per Serving:**

- Calories 230
- Fat 9 g
- Saturated fat 2 g
- Carbohydrates 7 g
- Fiber 0 g
- Protein 28 g
- Cholesterol 66 mg
- Sugars 3 g
- Sodium 341 mg
- Potassium 549 mg

# Lemon Garlic Salmon Pasta

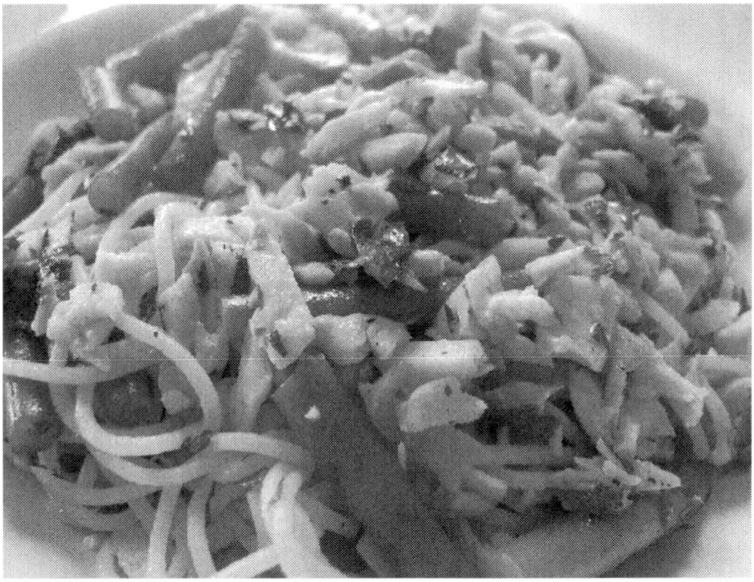

If you're craving for pasta but you're bored with the usual carbonara or Bolognese that you always eat, try this recipe. This one infused linguine with lemon garlic flavors, and umami from salmon.

**Serving size:** 4

**Preparation Cooking Time:** 20 minutes

**Ingredients:**

- 5 tablespoons olive oil
- 5 cloves garlic, crushed and minced
- ¼ teaspoon crushed red pepper
- 1 tablespoon lemon juice
- 1 teaspoon lemon zest
- 1 teaspoon anchovy paste
- 1 cup salmon, cooked and flaked
- 3 tablespoons parsley, chopped
- Salt to taste
- 4 cups cooked whole wheat linguine

**Instructions:**

1. In a pan over medium heat, pour the oil and stir in the garlic, red pepper, lemon juice, lemon zest, and anchovy paste.

2. Cook for 3 minutes.

3. Add ½ cup water, parsley and salt.

4. Cook while stirring for 2 minutes.

5. Top with the salmon flakes.

**Nutrients per Serving:**

- Calories 473
- Fat 23 g
- Saturated fat 3 g
- Carbohydrates 49 g
- Fiber 6 g
- Protein 20 g
- Cholesterol 25 mg
- Sugars 4 g
- Sodium 395 mg
- Potassium 513 mg

# Potato Curry with Chickpeas

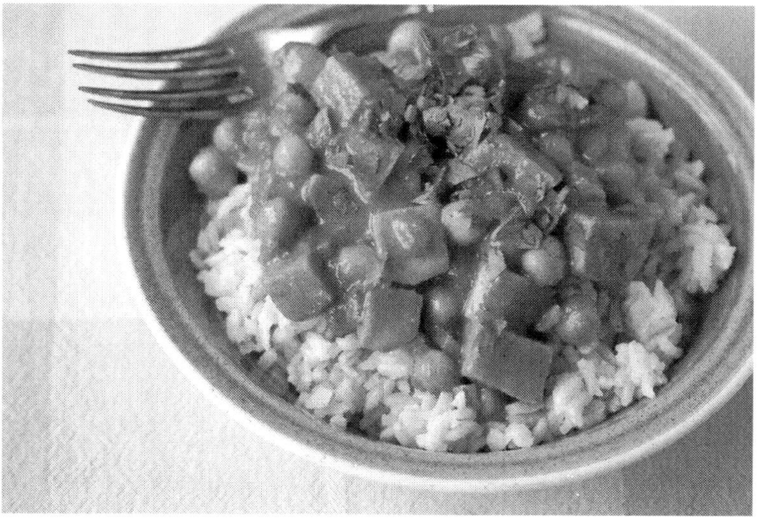

Even if you don't have chicken or fish, you can enjoy your favorite curry dish. This recipe makes use of potatoes, as well as chickpeas and green peas. This will surely satisfy your craving.

**Serving size:** 4

**Preparation Cooking Time:** 30 minutes

**Ingredients:**

- 1 lb. potatoes, sliced into cubes
- 3 tablespoons vegetable oil
- 1 onion, diced
- 4 cloves garlic, crushed and minced
- 2 teaspoons curry powder
- Salt to taste
- ¼ teaspoon cayenne pepper
- 14 oz. diced tomatoes
- 1 cup water, divided
- 15 oz. reduced-sodium chickpeas, rinsed and drained
- 1 cup peas
- ½ teaspoon garam masala

**Instructions:**

1. Fill your pot with water.

2. Add a steamer basket inside.

3. Steam the potatoes for 8 to 10 minutes.

4. Remove from heat and set aside.

5. Pour the oil in a pan over medium heat.

6. Cook the onion for 4 minutes.

7. Stir in the garlic and season with the salt, cayenne and curry powder.

8. Cook for 1 minute.

9. Add the tomatoes and juice and cook for 2 minutes.

10. Move the tomato mixture to a food processor.

11. Cook the potatoes and the rest of the ingredients in the tomato mixture.

12. Simmer for 5 minutes.

**Nutrients per Serving:**

- Calories 321
- Fat 12 g
- Saturated fat 1 g
- Carbohydrates 46 g
- Fiber 9 g
- Protein 9 g
- Cholesterol 0 mg
- Sugars 7 g
- Sodium 533 mg
- Potassium 796 mg

# Herbed Steak

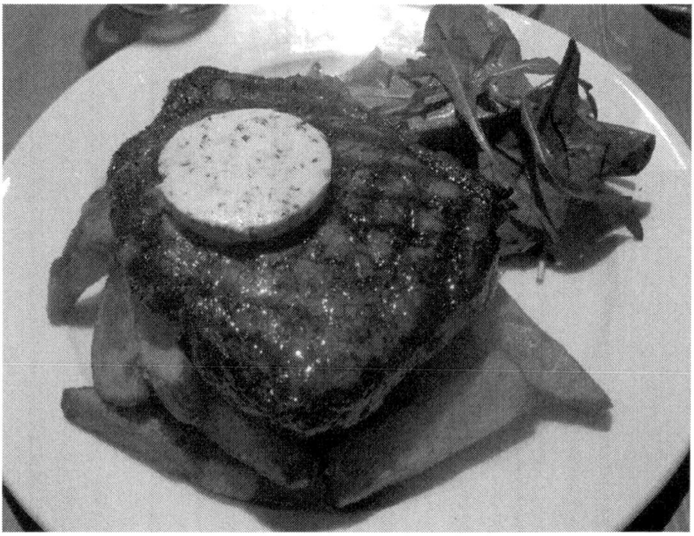

A dinner that will only take you 20 minutes or less to whip up! This is made extra special by searing the herbed steak in the pan and cooking the escarole in the same pan.

**Serving size:** 4

**Preparation Cooking Time:** 20 minutes

**Ingredients:**

- 1 lb. sirloin steak
- Salt and pepper to taste
- 2 tablespoons vegetable oil
- 1 sprig rosemary
- 5 sprigs thyme
- 3 sprigs sage
- 4 cloves garlic, crushed
- 16 cups escarole, chopped

**Instructions:**

1. Rub all both sides of the steak with the salt and pepper.

2. Put the pan over medium high heat.

3. Cook the steak for 3 minutes.

4. Flip and drizzle with the oil.

5. Top with the fresh herb sprigs and garlic.

6. Cook for 4 minutes.

7. Transfer to a plate and cover with foil to keep warm.

8. Add the escarole to your pan and season with the salt and pepper.

9. Cook for 2 minutes.

10. Serve the steak with the escarole.

**Nutrients per Serving:**

- Calories 244
- Fat 12 g
- Saturated fat 2 g
- Carbohydrates 10 g
- Fiber 8 g
- Protein 26 g
- Cholesterol 59 mg
- Sugars 1 g
- Sodium 394 mg
- Potassium 1111 mg

# Turkey Kebab with Carrot Side

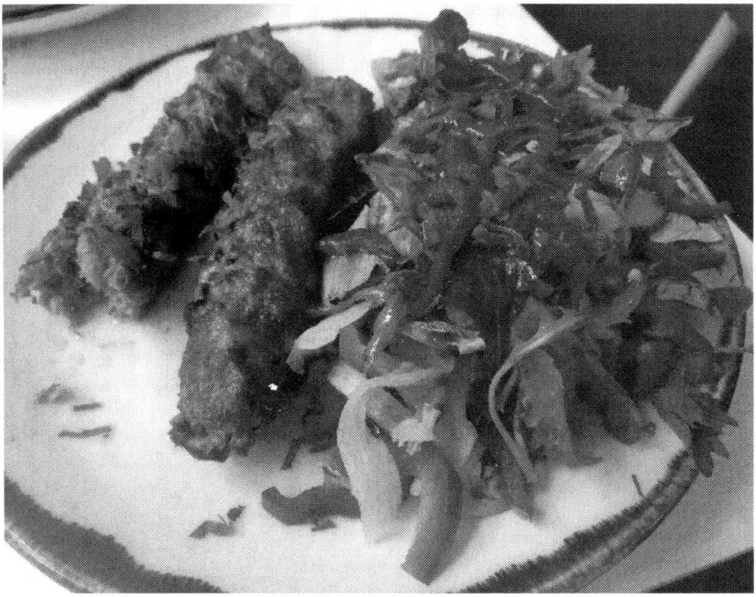

This turkey kebab is bursting with flavor thanks to the herbs and spices. To round up the flavor, serve it with salad made with radish and carrot.

**Serving size:** 4

**Preparation Cooking Time:** 6 hours and 15 minutes

**Ingredients:**

**Kebab:**

- 1 cup plain yogurt
- 3 tablespoons lime juice
- 2 teaspoons lime zest
- 1 tablespoon ginger, minced
- 1 tablespoon garlic, minced
- 1 chili pepper, chopped
- 1 teaspoon ground cumin
- ½ teaspoon ground coriander
- 2 teaspoons paprika
- ½ teaspoon ground cardamom
- ¼ teaspoon cayenne pepper
- 2 lb. turkey tenderloin, cubed

**Salad:**

- 2 scallions, chopped
- ½ cup radishes, shredded
- 1½ cups carrot, shredded
- ½ cup raisins
- Salad Dressing
- ⅓ cup plain yogurt
- 1 tablespoon honey
- 1 tablespoon lime juice
- ¼ teaspoon lime zest
- ¼ teaspoon ground coriander

**Instructions:**

1. In a bowl, combine all the kebab ingredients except the turkey.

2. Mix well.

3. Marinate the turkey cubes in the mixture for 4 hours, covered in the refrigerator.

4. Combine the scallions, radishes, carrots and raisins in a bowl.

5. Toss in the combination of the salad dressing ingredients.

6. Chill in the refrigerator for 1 hour.

7. Thread the turkey cubes into skewers.

8. Grill around 15 minutes, turning once or twice.

9. Serve with the carrot and radish salad.

**Nutrients per Serving:**

- Calories 346
- Fat 3 g
- Saturated fat 1 g
- Carbohydrates 34 g
- Fiber 1.7 g
- Protein 47 g
- Cholesterol 109 mg
- Sugars 24 g
- Sodium 100 mg
- Potassium 670 mg

# Breaded Flounder with Black Beans

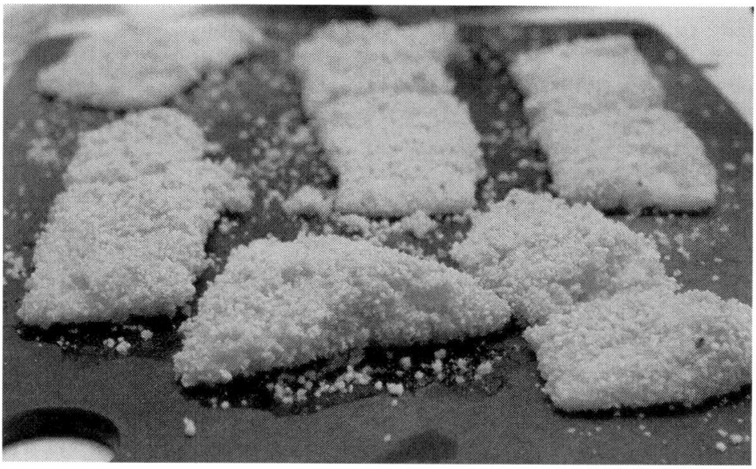

In this Mexican-inspired dish, we'll bread the fish with crushed tortilla chips, bake it until golden, and pair it with black beans.

**Serving size:** 4

**Preparation Cooking Time:** 40 minutes

**Ingredients:**

- Cooking spray
- 4 flounder fillets
- 4 oz. tortilla chips
- Pinch cayenne pepper
- 1 egg
- 15 oz. black beans (unsalted), rinsed and drained
- ¼ onion, chopped
- ½ cup green bell pepper, chopped
- ½ cup cherry tomatoes, sliced in half
- 2 tablespoons parsley, chopped
- 2 tablespoons oregano, chopped
- 2 teaspoons olive oil
- 1 tablespoon freshly squeezed lemon juice
- ¼ teaspoon ground cumin
- Salt to taste
- 1 oz. cheddar cheese

**Instructions:**

1. Preheat your oven to 425 degrees F.

2. Line your baking pan with foil.

3. Spray it with the oil.

4. Put the tortilla chips in the food processor.

5. Add the cayenne.

6. Process until crushed finely.

7. Transfer to a plate.

8. Add the egg to another plate. Beat the egg.

9. Coat the fish fillets with the egg and then dredge with tortilla chips.

10. Put the fish fillets on a baking pan.

11. Bake for 10 minutes.

12. In a bowl, combine the black beans, onion, bell pepper, tomatoes, parsley and oregano.

13. Stir in the olive oil, lemon juice, cumin, salt and pepper.

14. Place the fish on top of the beans and sprinkle top with the cheddar cheese.

**Nutrients per Serving:**

- Calories 361
- Fat 11 g
- Saturated fat 2 g
- Carbohydrates 35 g
- Fiber 8 g
- Protein 28 g
- Cholesterol 46 mg
- Sugars 3 g
- Sodium 401 mg
- Potassium 749 mg

# Irish Pork Roast

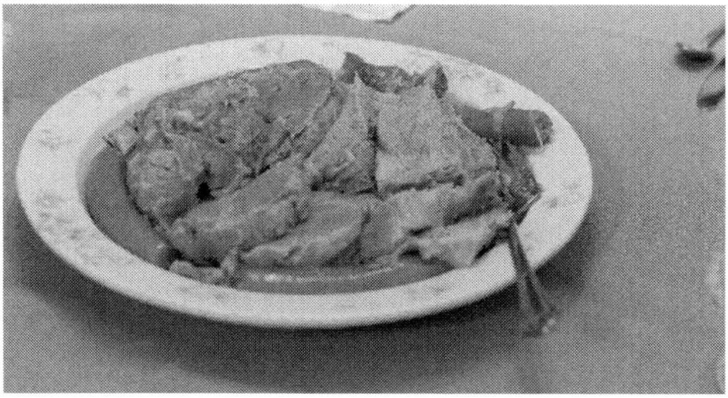

Want to do your pork roast differently? Roast it the Irish way. Here's the way to do it. It may not seem that simple but you'd know in the end all your effort would be worth it.

**Serving size:** 8

**Preparation Cooking Time:** 1 hour and 40 minutes

**Ingredients:**

- 1 lb. parsnips, sliced into cubes
- 2 lb. carrots, sliced into cubes
- 3 tablespoons olive oil, divided
- Salt and pepper to taste
- 2 teaspoons fresh thyme, divided
- 2 lb. pork loin roast (boneless)
- 1 cup dry hard cider
- 1 teaspoon honey
- Applesauce

**Instructions:**

1. Preheat your oven to 400 degrees F.

2. Place the parsnips and carrots in your bowl.

3. Coat with half of the oil and season with the salt, pepper and thyme.

4. Spread the mixture on a baking pan.

5. Rub the pork with the remaining oil and season with salt and pepper.

6. Place the pork roast on top of the carrots and parsnips.

7. Roast for 65 minutes.

8. Transfer the pork to a plate.

9. Stir in the cider and honey into the veggies.

10. Put on the stove and cook for 3 minutes.

11. Serve the pork roast with the veggies and applesauce.

**Nutrients per Serving:**

- Calories 272
- Fat 9 g
- Saturated fat 2 g
- Carbohydrates 23 g
- Fiber 6 g
- Protein 24 g
- Cholesterol 61 mg
- Sugars 10 g
- Sodium 327 mg
- Potassium 887 mg

# Trout in Lemon Butter Sauce

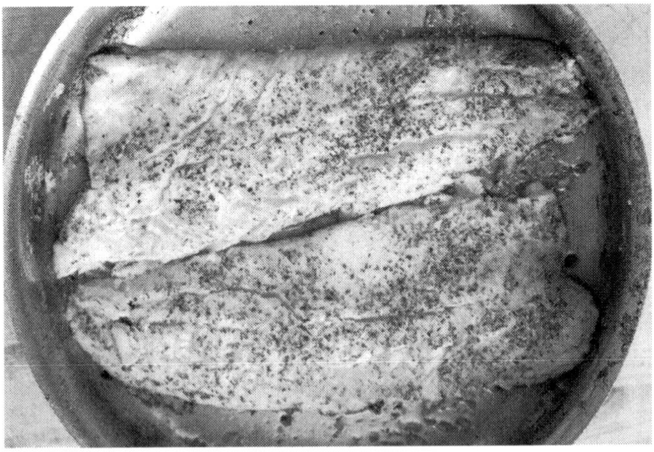

For something quick and easy, try this fish fillet recipe. In this recipe, you'll be coating the fish fillet with lemon glaze and serve it with leafy greens.

**Serving size:** 4

**Preparation Cooking Time:** 25 minutes

**Ingredients:**

- 4 oz. fish fillets
- Salt and pepper to taste
- ¼ cup low-fat milk
- ¼ cup whole-wheat flour
- 1 tablespoon olive oil
- 1 tablespoon shallot, chopped
- 2 tablespoons low-sodium chicken broth
- 1 tablespoon freshly squeezed lemon juice
- 1 tablespoon butter
- 1 tablespoon fresh parsley

**Instructions:**

1. Season the fish with salt and pepper.

2. Pour the milk in a dish.

3. Put the flour in another.

4. Dip each of the fish fillet into the milk, and then coat it with flour.

5. Pour the oil into a pan over medium heat.

6. Cook the fish for 3 to 4 minutes per side.

7. Transfer to a plate.

8. Add the rest of the ingredients in the pan.

9. Serve the fish with the wilted greens and pour the sauce on top.

**Nutrients per Serving:**

- Calories 240
- Fat 12 g
- Saturated fat 3 g
- Carbohydrates 7 g
- Fiber 1 g
- Protein 25 g
- Cholesterol 71 mg
- Sugars 1 g
- Sodium 173 mg
- Potassium 491 mg

# Cinnamon Pork Tenderloin with Caramelized Onions

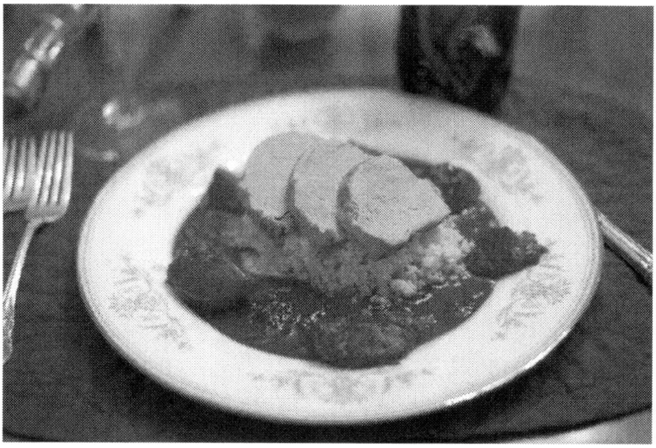

Pork tenderloin coated with cinnamon and all spice rub and served with peas, couscous and almonds.

**Serving size:** 4

**Preparation Cooking Time:** 2 hours and 10 minutes

**Ingredients:**

- ¼ teaspoon ground allspice
- ½ teaspoon ground cinnamon
- Salt and pepper to taste
- 1 lb. pork tenderloin
- 2 teaspoons olive oil, divided
- Cooking spray
- 1 cup onion, chopped
- ¼ cup orange juice
- 2 teaspoons cornstarch
- 2 teaspoons granulated sugar
- 2 tablespoons low-sodium soy sauce
- ½ teaspoon orange zest
- 2 cups couscous, cooked
- ¼ cup almonds, toasted and slivered
- ½ cup peas

**Instructions:**

1. Mix the allspice, cinnamon, salt and pepper in a bowl.

2. Rub the meat with this mixture.

3. Pour the oil into a pan over medium heat.

4. Cook the pork for 3 minutes per side.

5. Spray your slow cooker with oil.

6. Transfer the pork into the slow cooker.

7. Drop the remaining oil to the same pan.

8. Cook the onion for 4 minutes.

9. Place the onion on top of the pork.

10. Pour the orange juice into the pan.

11. Cover the pot and set it to low.

12. Cook for 2 hours.

13. Transfer the pork to a cutting board and slice.

14. Stir the cornstarch and sugar into the soy sauce.

15. Add the orange zest. Mix well.

16. Stir this mixture into the pot.

17. Cover the pot and cook for 15 more minutes.

18. In a bowl, combine the rest of the ingredients.

19. Serve the pork with the couscous mixture.

**Nutrients per Serving:**

- Calories 340
- Fat 10 g
- Saturated fat 2 g
- Carbohydrates 32 g
- Fiber 4 g
- Protein 29 g
- Cholesterol 71 mg
- Sugars 7 g
- Sodium 408 mg
- Potassium 651 mg

# Tofu in Peanut Sauce

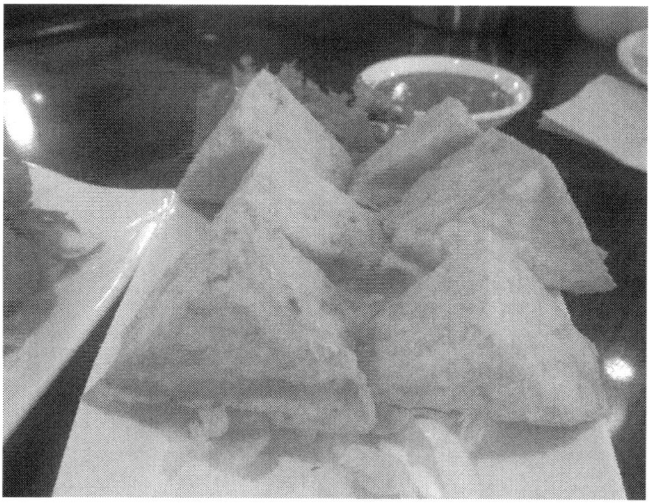

If you have your leftover rice from last night's dinner, this is one way to make good use of it. This stir-fried tofu with snow peas is also a good option when you're busy on a weeknight but want something delicious and filling.

**Serving size:** 4

**Preparation Cooking Time:** 30 minutes

**Ingredients:**

- 3 tablespoons rice vinegar
- ¼ cup peanut butter
- 2 teaspoons brown sugar
- 2 tablespoons reduced-sodium soy sauce
- 1 teaspoon hot sauce
- 14 oz. firm tofu, sliced into cubes
- 4 teaspoons vegetable oil, divided
- 3 cloves garlic, crushed and minced
- 2 tablespoons ginger, grated
- 2 cups snow peas
- 14 oz. frozen stir-fry veggies
- 4 tablespoons peanuts (unsalted), toasted
- 2 cups cooked rice

**Instructions:**

1. Prepare the peanut sauce by mixing the vinegar, peanut butter, brown sugar, soy sauce and hot sauce. Set aside.

2. Pour half of the oil into a pan over medium heat.

3. Cook the tofu until golden.

4. Drain on a plate lined with paper towel.

5. Pour the remaining oil to the pan.

6. Add the garlic, ginger, snow peas and frozen vegetables.

7. Stir fry for 4 minutes.

8. Stir in the sauce.

9. Put the tofu back to the pan.

10. Cook for 30 seconds, stirring frequently.

11. Serve on top of the rice and sprinkle with the peanuts.

**Nutrients per Serving:**

- Calories 514
- Fat 27 g
- Saturated fat 4 g
- Carbohydrates 49 g
- Fiber 7 g
- Protein 22 g
- Cholesterol 0 mg
- Sugars 12 g
- Sodium 376 mg
- Potassium 319 mg

# Baked Fish with Potatoes Mushrooms

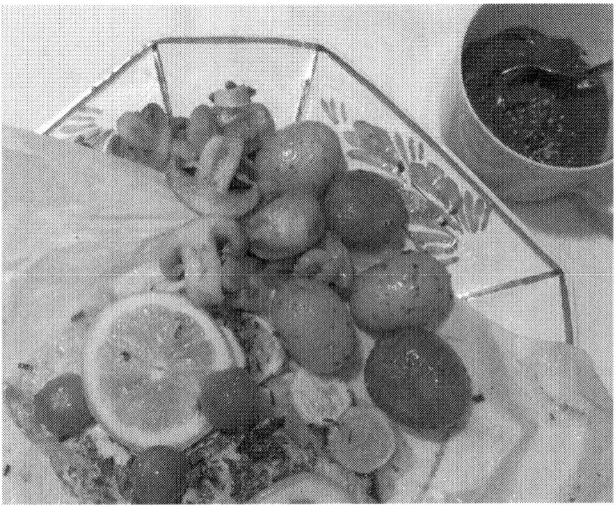

Only 15 active preparation time is needed to whip up this great meal that's inspired by southern French cuisine. If you don't have cod, you can also make use of other fish fillets like grouper or halibut.

**Serving size:** 4

**Preparation Cooking Time:** 1 hour

**Ingredients:**

- 1 lb. mushroomed, sliced
- 1 lb. potatoes, sliced into cubes
- 2 tablespoons olive oil, divided
- Salt and pepper to taste
- 2 cloves garlic, sliced
- 4 cod fillets
- 4 tablespoons freshly squeezed lemon juice
- 1 teaspoon herbes de Provence

**Instructions:**

1. Preheat your oven to 425 degrees F.

2. In a baking pan, toss the mushrooms and potatoes in half of the oil and season with the salt and pepper.

3. Bake in the oven for 40 minutes.

4. Stir and add the garlic.

5. Put the fish fillets on top.

6. Drizzle with the remaining oil and lemon juice.

7. Season with the herbes de Provence.

8. Bake for 15 minutes.

**Nutrients per Serving:**

- Calories 276
- Fat 9 g
- Saturated fat 1 g
- Carbohydrates 25 g
- Fiber 3 g
- Protein 24 g
- Cholesterol 49 mg
- Sugars 3 g
- Sodium 219 mg
- Potassium 1435 mg

# Shrimp Boil

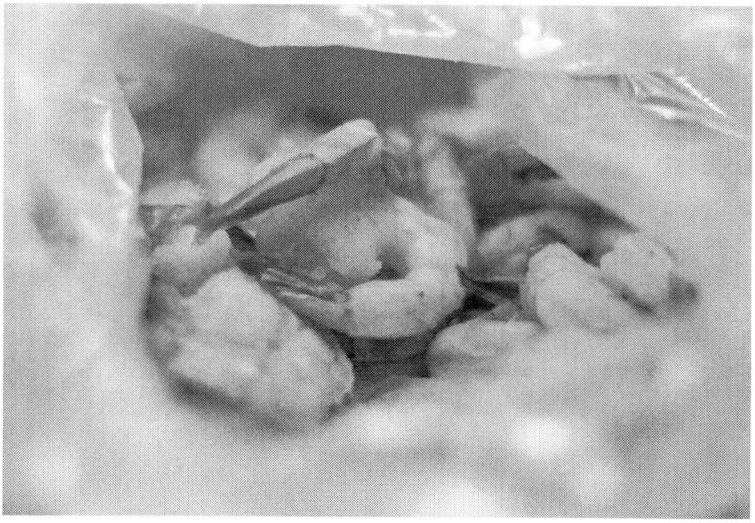

Here's an irresistible dish that you'd want to serve when you're having friends over. Your friends will adore the combination of corn, shrimp and sausages.

**Serving size:** 4

**Preparation Cooking Time:** 40 minutes

**Ingredients:**

- 3 tablespoons freshly squeezed lemon juice
- ¼ cup Old Bay seasoning
- 3 qt. water
- 8 oz. baby potatoes, sliced in half
- 8 oz. shrimp
- 2 ears corn, cut in half
- 1 leek, chopped
- 5 oz. chicken sausage, sliced

**Instructions:**

1. Stir the lemon juice and Old Bay seasoning into the water in a pot.

2. Bring to a boil.

3. Add the baby potatoes and cook for 15 minutes.

4. Stir in the shrimp, corn, leek and sausage.

5. Cook for 6 minutes.

6. Pour the sauce over the shrimp mixture and serve.

**Nutrients per Serving:**

- Calories 202
- Fat 5 g
- Saturated fat 1 g
- Carbohydrates 22 g
- Fiber 2 g
- Protein 19 g
- Cholesterol 109 mg
- Sugars 5 g
- Sodium 582 mg
- Potassium 568 mg

# Lemon Pepper Salmon

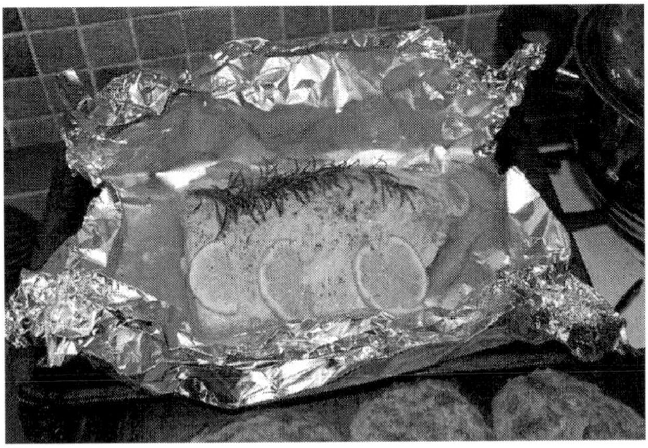

This dish is too easy to cook that there's a good chance that you're going to regularly include this in your menu. You'd love how wrapping the fish seals in all the flavors and moisture and makes cleanup simpler.

**Serving size:** 4

**Preparation Cooking Time:** 25 minutes

**Ingredients:**

- 4 salmon fillets
- Salt to taste
- 2 tablespoons butter (unsalted)
- 1 lemon, sliced thinly
- 1 teaspoon lemon pepper
- Parsley, chopped

**Instructions:**

1. Preheat your grill.

2. Place the salmon fillets on top of foil sheet.

3. Top each fillet with salt, butter, lemon slice, lemon pepper and parsley.

4. Wrap the fish with the foil.

5. Place on the grill and cook for 10 minutes.

6. Flip and cook for another 5 minutes.

**Nutrients per Serving:**

- Calories 256
- Fat 12 g
- Saturated fat 5 g
- Carbohydrates 1 g
- Fiber 1 g
- Protein 34 g
- Cholesterol 95 mg
- Sugars 1 g
- Sodium 165 mg
- Potassium 653 mg

# Caprese Salad

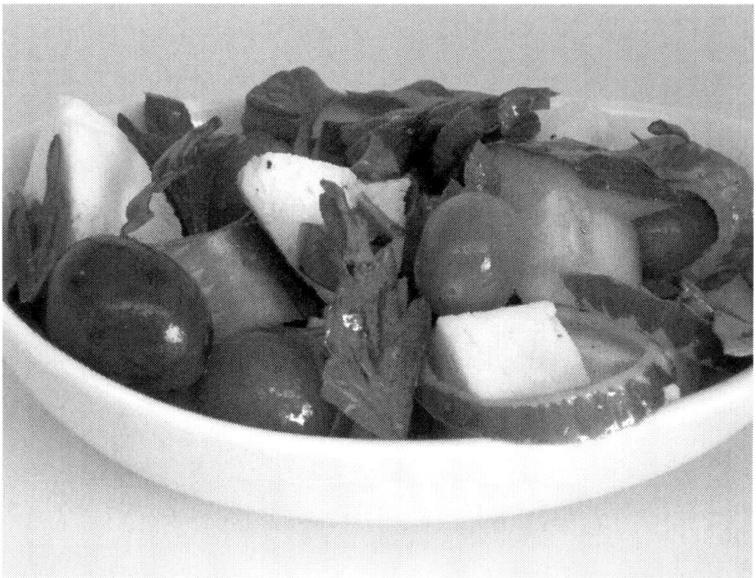

Do you love Caprese salad? If yes, then you'll also adore its sandwich version. This toast is topped with basil, tomatoes, mozzarella, and avocado.

**Serving size:** 4

**Preparation Cooking Time:** 10 minutes

**Ingredients:**

- 4 slices whole-wheat bread
- 1 avocado, sliced
- Pepper to taste
- 2 tablespoons freshly squeezed lemon juice
- 8 basil leaves
- 1 tomato, sliced
- 4 slices mozzarella cheese
- 4 teaspoons balsamic vinegar

**Instructions:**

1. Toast the bread for 3 minutes.

2. In medium bowl, mash the avocado and stir in the pepper and lemon juice.

3. Spread this mixture on top of the bread.

4. Top with the basil, tomatoes and mozzarella.

5. Drizzle with the balsamic vinegar.

**Nutrients per Serving:**

- Calories 322
- Fat 21 g
- Saturated fat 5 g
- Carbohydrates 25 g
- Fiber 9 g
- Protein 11 g
- Cholesterol 20 mg
- Sugars 5 g
- Sodium 225 mg
- Potassium 735 mg

# Chicken Oat Sandwich

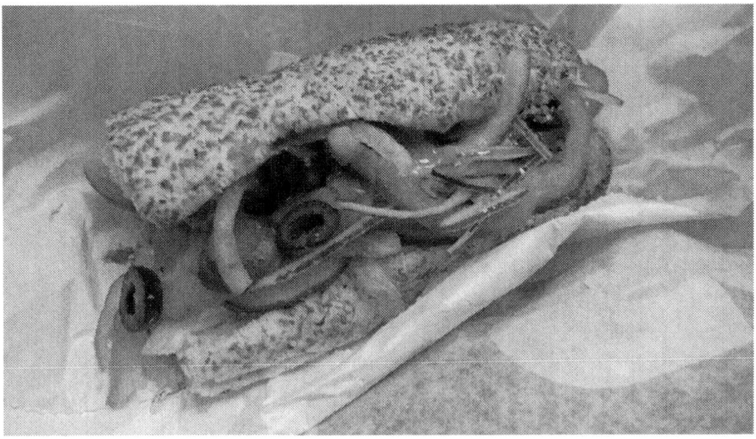

You might never have thought about using oats for your sandwich, but this is a definite must-try. The oats lend interesting texture to this sandwich that's stuffed with bacon, chicken, lettuce, tomatoes and onion.

**Serving size:** 4

**Preparation Cooking Time:** 45 minutes

**Ingredients:**

- 2 tablespoons low-fat mayonnaise
- ½ teaspoon lime juice
- ½ teaspoon sugar
- 1 teaspoon low-sodium chipotle chili pepper in adobo sauce, chopped
- Cooking spray
- 1 lb. chicken breast fillet (skinless), sliced
- 1 tablespoon water
- ¼ cup plain yogurt
- ¼ cup rolled oats
- ½ cup breadcrumbs
- 3 tablespoons dried cherries, chopped
- 4 whole-wheat bread slices
- 8 lettuce leaves
- 8 slices reduced-sodium bacon, cooked
- 4 tomato slices
- 4 onion rings

**Instructions:**

1. In a bowl, mix the mayo, lime juice, sugar, and chipotle chili pepper. Set aside.

2. Preheat your oven to 425 degrees F.

3. Cover the baking pan with foil.

4. Coat it with cooking spray.

5. In another bowl, mix the water and yogurt.

6. In the third bowl, combine the oats, breadcrumbs and cherries.

7. Dip the chicken in the first bowl, and then in the second bowl.

8. Arrange in a single layer on a baking sheet.

9. Bake for 20 minutes.

10. Spread the mayo mixture on the bread slices.

11. Place the lettuce leaves on top.

12. Top with the baked chicken, bacon, tomato and onion ring.

13. Place another bread slice on top.

**Nutrients per Serving:**

- Calories 361
- Fat 9 g
- Saturated fat 2 g
- Carbohydrates 36 g
- Fiber 7 g
- Protein 36 g
- Cholesterol 80 mg
- Sugars 9 g
- Sodium 567 mg
- Potassium 448 mg

# Hummus Sandwich with Roasted Veggies

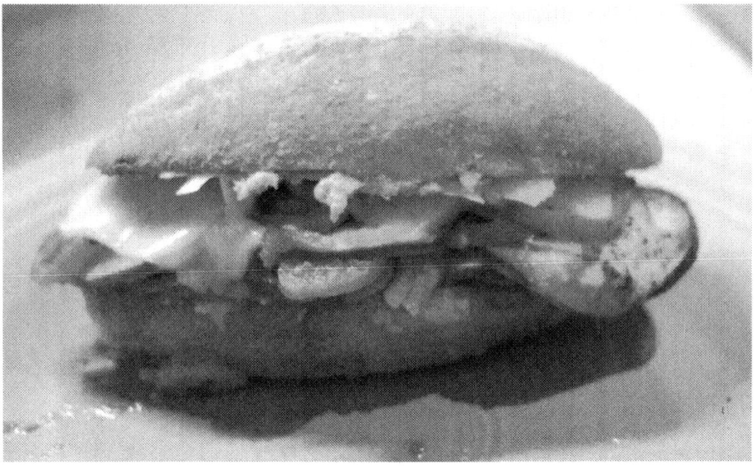

You and your lovely family will surely be delighted with this simple but appetizing snack idea. Hummus spread on whole wheat bread slices and topped with flavorful roasted veggies.

**Serving size:** 2

**Preparation Cooking Time:** 40 minutes

**Ingredients:**

- ¼ cup bell pepper strips
- ¼ cup squash, sliced
- ¼ cup eggplant, sliced
- 2 teaspoons olive oil
- 2 slices whole-wheat bread
- 4 tablespoons hummus
- 1 cup spinach leaves, chopped
- 4 basil leaves, chopped
- 2 teaspoons sunflower seeds (unsalted)

**Instructions:**

1. Preheat your oven to 350 degrees F.

2. Toss the bell pepper, squash and eggplant in olive oil.

3. Transfer to a baking dish.

4. Bake in the oven for 20 to 25 minutes.

5. Toast the bread slices and spread the hummus on top.

6. Top each with the spinach and roasted vegetables.

7. Sprinkle with the chopped basil and sunflower seeds.

**Nutrients per Serving:**

- Calories 270
- Fat 15 g
- Saturated fat 2 g
- Carbohydrates 27 g
- Fiber 8 g
- Protein 11 g
- Cholesterol 0 mg
- Sugars 3 g
- Sodium 394 mg
- Potassium 655 mg

# Mushroom Ricotta Open Face Sandwich

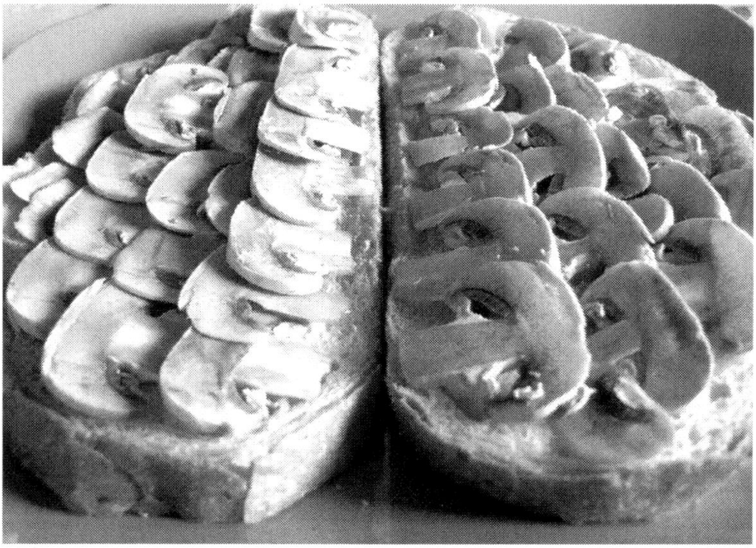

There's no denying that the combination of cheese and mushroom is always a good idea. If you want a quick and healthy snack without the fuss, use this foolproof combination on your sandwich.

**Serving size:** 2

**Preparation Cooking Time:** 15 minutes

**Ingredients:**

- 2 teaspoons olive oil
- 1 cup mushrooms, sliced
- 2 tablespoons lemon juice
- 2 teaspoons lemon zest
- 1 teaspoon garlic, minced
- ½ cup ricotta cheese
- 2 slices whole wheat bread
- 1 tablespoon balsamic vinegar

**Instructions:**

1. Pour the oil into a pan over medium heat.

2. Cook the mushrooms for 10 minutes.

3. In a bowl, combine the lemon juice, lemon zest, garlic and ricotta cheese.

4. Spread this mixture on top of the bread slices.

5. Arrange the mushrooms on top and drizzle with the balsamic vinegar.

**Nutrients per Serving:**

- Calories 219
- Fat 10 g
- Saturated fat 4 g
- Carbohydrates 20 g
- Fiber 2 g
- Protein 12 g
- Cholesterol 19 mg
- Sugars 4 g
- Sodium 194 mg
- Potassium 349 mg

# Chicken Curry Sandwich

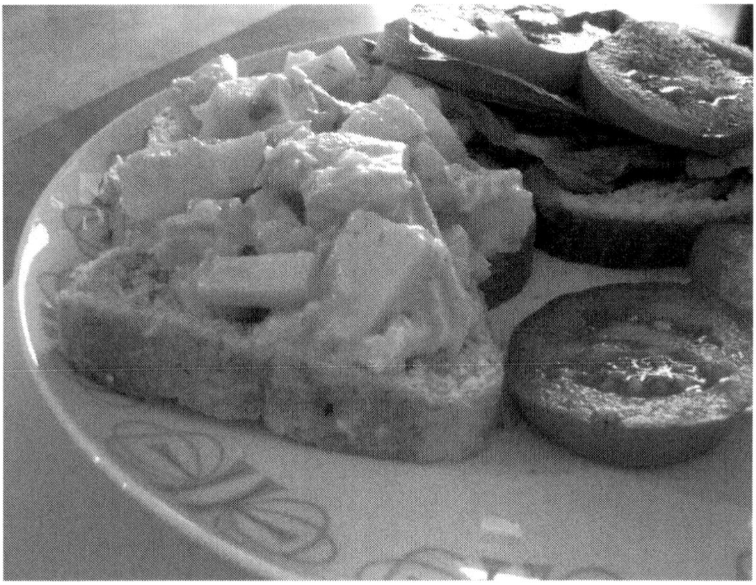

This gives a unique twist to your favorite chicken salad sandwich. It is spruced up with the addition of curry powder, cumin, raisins and cashews.

**Serving size:** 2

**Preparation Cooking Time:** 10 minutes

**Ingredients:**

- 2 slices whole wheat bread
- 4 oz. canned chicken flakes in water, drained
- ½ cup carrot, shredded
- 2 tablespoons olive oil
- 2 tablespoons plain yogurt
- 6 cashews, chopped
- 4 raisins, chopped
- ¼ teaspoon ground cumin
- ½ teaspoon curry powder
- Salt and pepper to taste
- Cilantro, chopped

**Instructions:**

1. Toast the bread slices.

2. In your bowl, mix all the ingredients except the cilantro.

3. Spread the mixture on top of the bread.

4. Garnish with the cilantro.

**Nutrients per Serving:**

- Calories 326
- Fat 19 g
- Saturated fat 3 g
- Carbohydrates 18 g
- Fiber 3 g
- Protein 21 g
- Cholesterol 48 mg
- Sugars 4 g
- Sodium 306 mg
- Potassium 329 mg

# Bagel with Veggies Cream Cheese

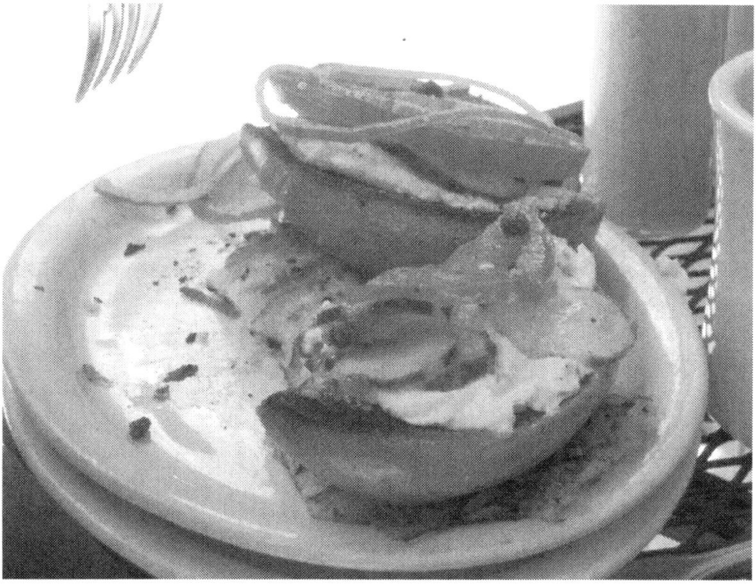

Here's a bagel sandwich that would appeal to almost anyone. It turns out the avocado and other veggies in this recipe go so well together with cream cheese and bagel that you simply resist this wonderful snack idea.

**Serving size:** 4

**Preparation Cooking Time:** 30 minutes

**Ingredients:**

- ½ cup cream cheese (unsalted)
- Salt and pepper to taste
- 1 tablespoon dried dill
- 4 whole wheat bagels
- 4 avocado slices
- 8 cucumber slices
- 1 red bell pepper, sliced and roasted into strips
- 1 onion, sliced into rings

**Instructions:**

1. Mix the cream cheese, salt, pepper and dill in a bowl.

2. Spread each bagel with this mixture.

3. Top with the slices of avocado and cucumber, red bell pepper strips and onion rings.

**Nutrients per Serving:**

- Calories 222
- Fat 8 g
- Saturated fat 3 g
- Carbohydrates 31 g
- Fiber 5 g
- Protein 9 g
- Cholesterol 13 mg
- Sugars 1 g
- Sodium 301 mg
- Potassium 550 mg

# Shrimp Tacos

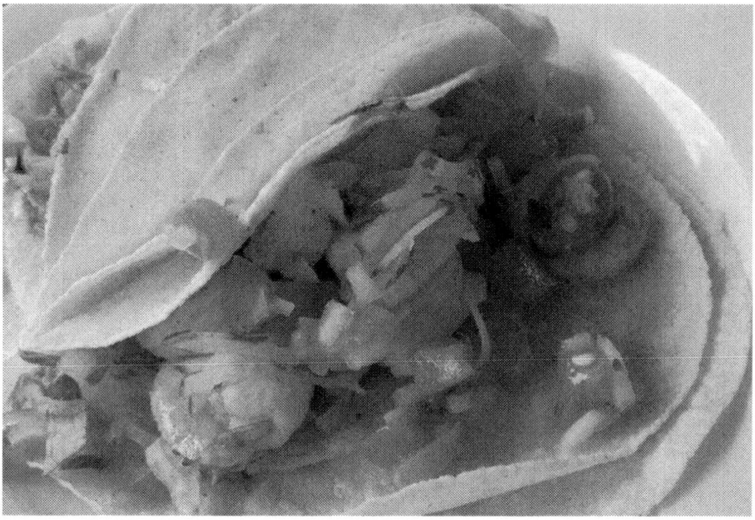

This shrimp taco recipe is perfect for last-minute snacks or when you just don't have the patience to go through extensive kitchen preparation. Shrimp takes only a few minutes to cook.

**Serving size:** 2

**Preparation Cooking Time:** 20 minutes

**Ingredients:**

- ½ avocado
- 1 garlic, grated
- Salt to taste
- ½ tablespoon lemon juice
- ½ lb. shrimp, peeled and deveined
- 1 tablespoon Cajun seasoning (unsalted)
- 4 corn tortillas
- 1 cup lettuce, chopped
- ¼ cup pico de gallo
- ¼ cup cilantro

**Instructions:**

1. Preheat your grill.

2. Mash the avocado in a bowl.

3. Stir in the garlic, salt and lemon juice.

4. Toss the peeled shrimp in the Cajun seasoning.

5. Thread each one into skewers.

6. Grill for 2 minutes per side.

7. Stuff the corn tortilla with the shrimp, avocado mixture, lettuce, pico de gallo and cilantro.

**Nutrients per Serving:**

- Calories 286
- Fat 1 g
- Saturated fat 7 g
- Carbohydrates 30 g
- Fiber 7 g
- Protein 24 g
- Cholesterol 159 mg
- Sugars 4 g
- Sodium 443 mg
- Potassium 662 mg

# Pork Fajitas

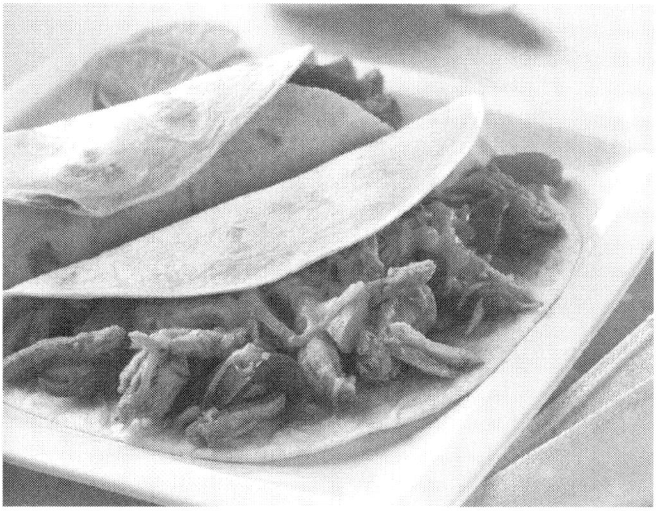

Fajita is a Mexican staple in which grilled meat is served in corn tortilla or taco. It is usually accompanied by tomatoes, cheese, sour cream, lettuce and beans. Most people use beef on their fajitas, but for this one, we opted to use pulled pork. Another thing that makes this recipe unique is the addition of mangoes.

**Serving size:** 2

**Preparation Cooking Time:** 5 hours and 50 minutes

**Ingredients:**

- 1 lb. pork shoulder roast, fat trimmed
- Salt and pepper to taste
- 2 teaspoons chili powder
- 1 cup water, divided
- ½ cup tomatillos, chopped
- 2 tablespoons onion, chopped
- 2 tablespoons jalapeño, chopped
- 1 tablespoon cilantro, chopped
- 1 tablespoon freshly squeezed lime juice
- 2 cloves garlic, crushed and minced
- 6 corn tortillas
- 6 tablespoons mango, chopped

**Instructions:**

1. Season the pork with the pepper, salt and chili powder.

2. Transfer to a slow cooker.

3. Pour half of the water into the pot.

4. Cover and set it to high.

5. Cook for 5 hours.

6. Transfer to a cutting board.

7. Let cool and then pull the meat into shreds. Set aside.

8. In a pan, combine the rest of the ingredients except the tortilla and mango.

9. Add the remaining water.

10. Cook for 15 minutes.

11. Top each tortilla with the pulled pork, salsa and chopped mango.

**Nutrients per Serving:**

- Calories 338
- Fat 10 g
- Saturated fat 3 g
- Carbohydrates 29 g
- Fiber 3 g
- Protein 32 g
- Cholesterol 92 mg
- Sugars 7 g
- Sodium 563 mg
- Potassium 761 mg

# Grilled Burger

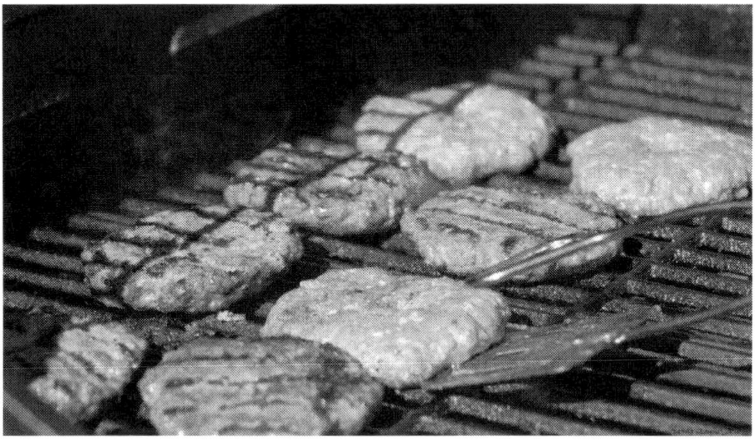

If you think this is just another burger recipe, you're wrong. This one is made a lot more special by adding scallions and carrots into the burger patty and spreading it with curry mustard sauce. It has an incredible flavor that will make you crave for it over and over.

**Serving size:** 4

**Preparation Cooking Time:** 35 minutes

**Ingredients:**

- ½ teaspoon curry powder
- ¼ cup Dijon mustard
- 1 lb. lean ground beef
- ¼ cup scallions, chopped
- ½ cup carrot, shredded
- ¼ cup breadcrumbs
- ¼ teaspoon dried Italian seasoning
- ¼ teaspoon garlic salt
- Pepper to taste
- 2 tablespoons milk
- 4 whole wheat burger buns
- Tomato slices
- Lettuce leaves

**Instructions:**

1. Combine the curry powder and mustard in a bowl and set aside.

2. In another bowl, mix all the ingredients except the buns, tomatoes and lettuce.

3. Mix well.

4. Form thick patties from the mixture.

5. Grill the burgers for 8 to 10 minutes per side.

6. Place the lettuce and burgers on the buns.

7. Top with the tomatoes.

8. Drizzle with the mustard sauce.

**Nutrients per Serving:**

- Calories 257
- Fat 9 g
- Saturated fat 4 g
- Carbohydrates 24 g
- Fiber 3 g
- Protein 20 g
- Cholesterol 54 mg
- Sugars 1 g
- Sodium 409 mg
- Potassium 541 mg

# Mini Pizza

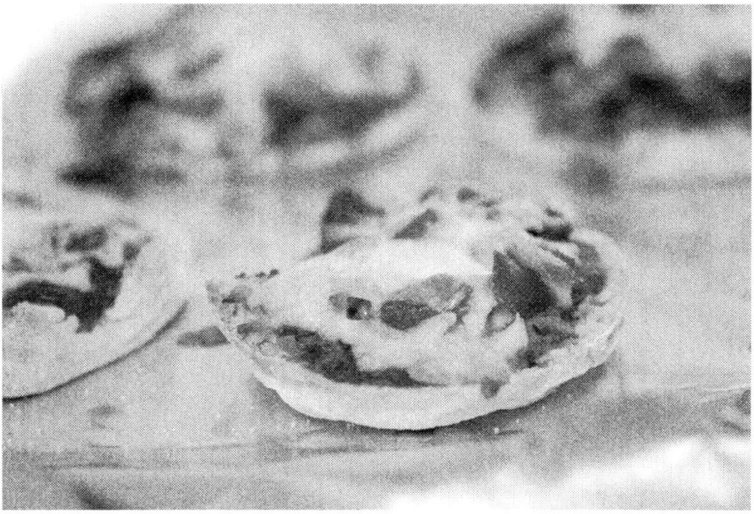

Here's another great snack idea that won't disappoint. It's mini pizza. It may be small in size, but it certainly doesn't lack in flavor and appeal. Instead of pizza dough, we make use of bread for this recipe.

**Serving size:** 8

**Preparation Cooking Time:** 20 minutes

**Ingredients:**

- 8 slices bread
- ½ cup tomato sauce (unsalted)
- ¼ teaspoon crushed red pepper
- 1 teaspoon dried Italian seasoning, crushed
- ½ cup red bell pepper, sliced into strips
- 3 oz. turkey sausage, cooked and crumbled
- ¾ cup mozzarella cheese

**Instructions:**

1. Preheat your oven to 400 degrees F.

2. Bake the bread in the oven for 5 minutes.

3. While waiting, mix the tomato sauce, red pepper and Italian seasoning.

4. Spread this mixture on top of the bread.

5. Top with the bell pepper strips and crumbled sausage.

6. Sprinkle the mozzarella cheese on top.

7. Bake until the cheese has melted.

**Nutrients per Serving:**

- Saturated fat 1 g
- Sugars 3 g
- Fat 4 g
- Calories 105
- Carbohydrates 13 g
- Fiber 3 g
- Protein 8 g
- Cholesterol 14 mg
- Sodium 256 mg
- Potassium 52 mg

# Green Beans Potato Salad

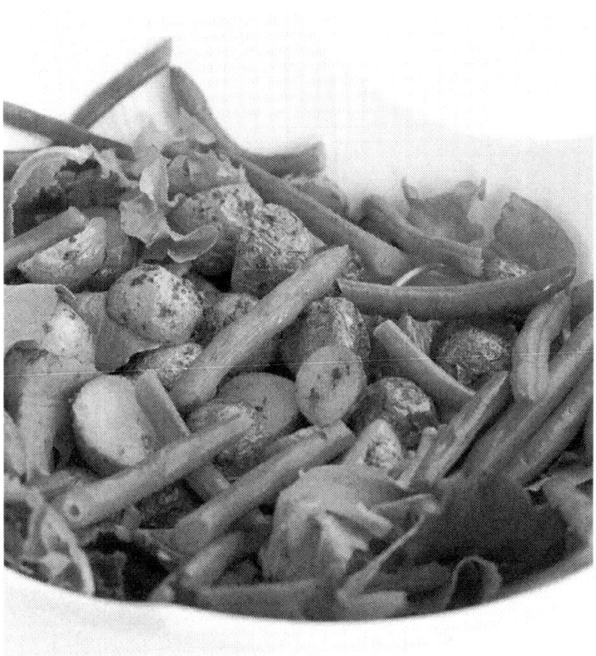

Can't decide whether to prepare green beans salad or potato salad? Why don't you make a combination of these two? Here's an awesome recipe that you should try. Making it more flavorful is the sprinkling of fresh chopped dill.

**Serving size:** 6

**Preparation Cooking Time:** 40 minutes

**Ingredients:**

**Dressing:**

- 3 tablespoons olive oil
- 1½ tablespoons white-wine vinegar
- ½ teaspoon Dijon mustard
- 1½ tablespoons freshly squeezed lemon juice
- 1 teaspoon lemon zest
- ¼ teaspoon honey
- Salt and pepper to taste
- 2 tablespoons fresh dill, chopped

**Salad:**

- 1½ lb. baby potatoes, sliced in half
- 2 cloves garlic, minced
- 12 oz. green beans, trimmed and sliced
- ½ cup shallot, chopped
- 2 tablespoons olive oil
- Dill sprigs

**Instructions:**

1. Combine all the dressing ingredients in a glass jar with lid.

2. Shake to blend well.

3. Prepare the salad by boiling garlic and potatoes in a pot with water.

4. Cook for 10 minutes.

5. Discard the garlic.

6. Soak the beans in the same pot and cook for 2 minutes.

7. Toss the beans and potatoes in the dressing.

8. Drizzle with the olive oil and sprinkle with the shallots.

9. Garnish with the dill sprigs before serving.

**Nutrients per Serving:**

- Calories 216
- Fat 12 g
- Saturated fat 2 g
- Carbohydrates 25 g
- Fiber 4 g
- Protein 4 g
- Cholesterol 0 mg
- Sugars 4 g
- Sodium 125 mg
- Potassium 648 mg

# Citrus Garden Salad

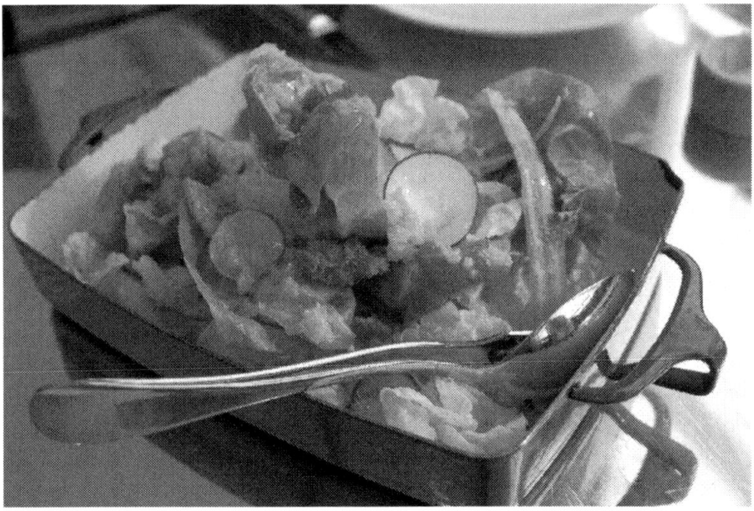

The colors are more than enough to entice you. Wait until you get a taste of this amazing salad recipe made with leafy greens, oranges, grapefruit and pomegranate seeds.

**Serving size:** 8

**Preparation Cooking Time:** 25 minutes

**Ingredients:**

- 5 tablespoons olive oil
- 3 tablespoons freshly squeezed lemon juice
- 2 teaspoons Dijon mustard
- 2 tablespoons honey
- 1 tablespoon shallot, minced
- 1 tablespoon fresh thyme, chopped
- Salt and pepper to taste
- 3 oranges, sliced into segments
- 1 grapefruit, sliced
- 4 cups salad greens
- ¼ cup pomegranate seeds

**Instructions:**

1. Prepare the perfect dressing by mixing the olive oil, lemon juice, mustard, honey, shallot, thyme, salt and pepper.

2. In a large salad bowl, toss the oranges, grapefruit and salad greens.

3. Pour the dressing over the salad and mix well.

4. Sprinkle the pomegranate seeds on top of the salad.

**Nutrients per Serving:**

- Calories 144
- Fat 9 g
- Saturated fat 1 g
- Carbohydrates 16 g
- Fiber 2 g
- Protein 1 g
- Cholesterol 0 mg
- Sugars 12 g
- Sodium 167 mg
- Potassium 195 mg

# Vegetable Salad

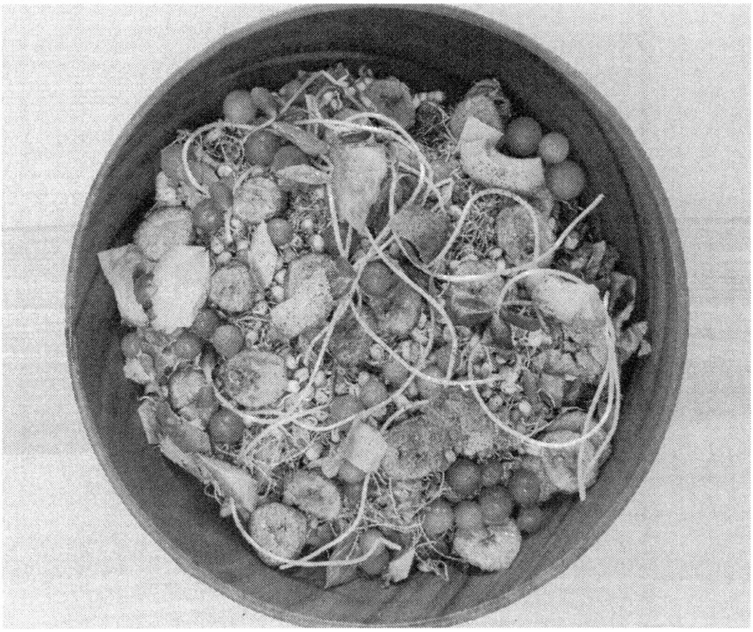

Prepare this healthy and satisfying salad for yourself or for your family. It's a quick combination of whatever veggies you have in your fridge or pantry.

**Serving size:** 6

**Preparation Cooking Time:** 15 minutes

**Ingredients:**

- ¼ cup olive oil
- ¼ cup vegetable oil
- 1 tablespoon cilantro, chopped
- 3 tablespoons freshly squeezed lime juice
- Salt and pepper to taste
- ½ cup baby potatoes, sliced and steamed
- ½ cup green beans, sliced and steamed
- ½ cup radishes, sliced
- ½ cup cucumbers, sliced
- ½ cup tomatoes, sliced
- 4 cups Romaine lettuce leaves, chopped
- 1 hard-boiled egg, sliced
- 1 onion, sliced into rings
- Feta cheese

**Instructions:**

1. Whisk the two oils in a bowl.

2. Add the cilantro, lime juice, pepper and salt.

3. Toss the veggies in half of this dressing.

4. Arrange the lettuce on a serving platter.

5. Top with the vegetables, egg slices, onion rings and feta cheese.

6. Drizzle the remaining dressing on top.

**Nutrients per Serving:**

- Calories 214
- Fat 20 g
- Saturated fat 2 g
- Carbohydrates 8 g
- Fiber 2 g
- Protein 3 g
- Cholesterol 31 mg
- Sugars 2 g
- Sodium 217 mg
- Potassium 680 mg

# Chicken Brussels Sprouts Salad

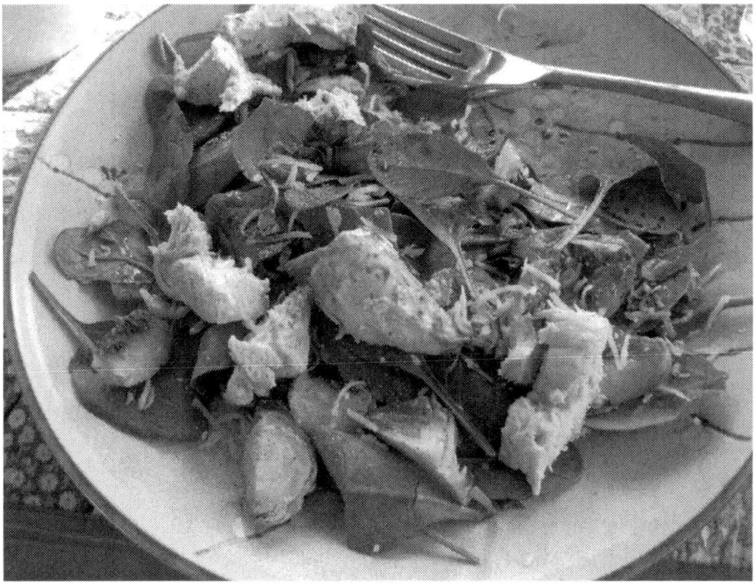

This is a good way to make use of leftover chicken from last night. Simply shred the chicken and toss it with leafy greens, Brussels sprouts and mushrooms, drizzle with vinaigrette, and that's it!

**Serving size:** 4

**Preparation Cooking Time:** 10 minutes

**Ingredients:**

- 6 tablespoons olive oil
- 1 tablespoon Dijon mustard
- 3 tablespoons red-wine vinegar
- 1½ tablespoons shallot, chopped
- Pepper to taste
- 2 teaspoons fresh thyme, chopped
- 4 cups arugula leaves
- 12 oz. chicken, cooked and shredded
- 4 cups Brussels sprouts, sliced
- 4 cups mushrooms
- 1 cup Parmesan cheese, grated

**Instructions:**

1. Prepare the dressing by blending the olive oil, mustard, vinegar, shallot, thyme and pepper.

2. Arrange the arugula leaves on a serving platter.

3. Top with the chicken, Brussels sprouts and mushrooms.

4. Drizzle the dressing on top.

5. Sprinkle the Parmesan cheese on top and serve.

**Nutrients per Serving:**

- Calories 432
- Fat 31 g
- Saturated fat 7 g
- Carbohydrates 15 g
- Fiber 5 g
- Protein 24 g
- Cholesterol 56 mg
- Sugars 6 g
- Sodium 533 mg
- Potassium 917 mg

# Pickled Beet Salad

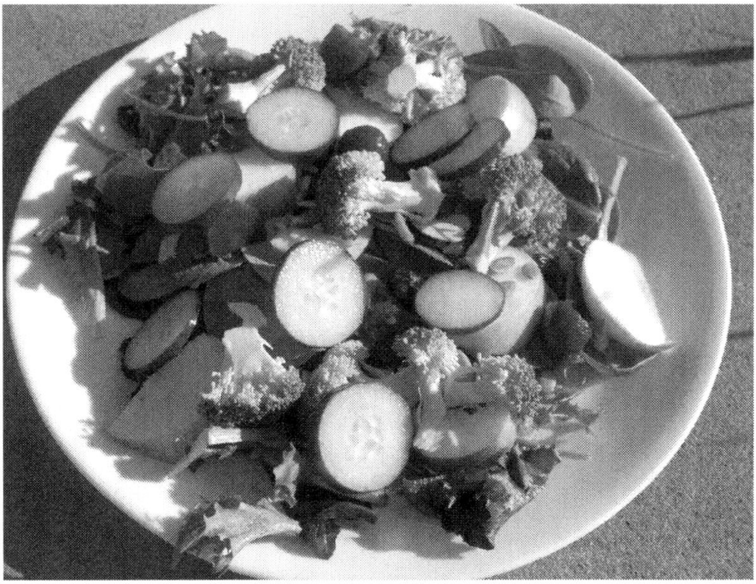

Have you tried making pickled beets? If not, you're missing a lot! Not only are these great as appetizers or sides, you can also use these to create a light and flavorful salad. Here's a recipe that you'd surely want to try.

**Serving size:** 4

**Preparation Cooking Time:** 1 hour and 5 minutes

**Ingredients:**

- ½ cup carrots, julienned
- ½ cup cucumber, julienned
- ½ cup radish, julienned
- 2 cups water
- ¼ cup rice vinegar
- ¾ cup sugar, divided
- 1 lb. beets, sliced into cubes
- 1 cup red-wine vinegar
- ¾ tablespoons ginger, grated
- ¾ teaspoons salt, divided
- 2 tablespoons sesame oil, divided
- 3 cups kale, chopped
- 1 clove garlic, crushed and minced

**Instructions:**

1. Put the julienned veggies in a bowl.

2. In a pan over medium heat, combine ¼ cup water with the rice vinegar and half of sugar.

3. Bring to a boil.

4. Pour this mixture over the veggies.

5. Let sit for 30 minutes.

6. Drain the water and then set aside.

7. Pour ½ cup water into a pot.

8. Add a steamer basket inside.

9. Steam the beets for 30 minutes.

10. Transfer to a bowl.

11. In a pan over medium heat, pour in the remaining water, remaining sugar, red wine vinegar, ginger and salt.

12. Remove from the stove.

13. Pour the mixture on top of the beets and marinate for 30 minutes.

14. In another pan, heat the sesame oil and add the kale and garlic.

15. Cook until wilted.

16. Transfer the kale to a food processor then blend until smooth.

17. Serve the beets and julienned veggies with the kale pesto.

**Nutrients per Serving:**

- Calories 127
- Fat 7 g
- Saturated fat 1 g
- Carbohydrates 14 g
- Fiber 3 g
- Protein 2 g
- Cholesterol 0 mg
- Sugars 10 g
- Sodium 191 mg
- Potassium 378 mg

# Creamy Celery Soup

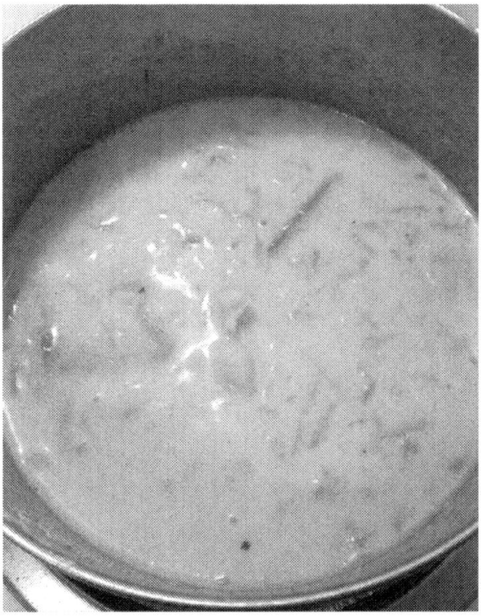

The combination of celery, fennel, tarragon and lemon makes this soup dish something that you'd want to serve when there's a special occasion.

**Serving size:** 8

**Preparation Cooking Time:** 30 minutes

**Ingredients:**

- 1 lb. celery
- 1 tablespoon olive oil
- 2 cups onions, chopped
- 4 cloves garlic, chopped
- 1 tablespoon fresh thyme, chopped
- ¾ teaspoon ground fennel seed
- 1 teaspoon lemon zest
- 4 cups chicken broth (unsalted)
- Salt and pepper to taste
- 1 tablespoon freshly squeezed lemon juice
- 2 tablespoons fresh tarragon leaves
- 2 cups fresh baby spinach
- ½ cup heavy cream

**Instructions:**

1. Separate the celery leaves from the stalks. Reserve the leaves for another use.

2. Chop the celery stalks finely.

3. Pour the oil in a pan over medium heat.

4. Cook the onion, garlic, celery stalks and thyme for 10 minutes.

5. Stir in the fennel and lemon zest.

6. Cook for 30 seconds, stirring frequently.

7. Pour in the broth and season with the salt.

8. Bring to a boil.

9. Stir in the lemon juice, tarragon and spinach.

10. Cook for 1 minute and then remove from heat.

11. Transfer to a food processor and blend.

12. Put the pureed soup back to the pot.

13. Heat through for 2 minutes.

14. Stir in the cream and season with the pepper.

**Nutrients per Serving:**

- Calories 141
- Fat 11 g
- Saturated fat 4 g
- Carbohydrates 8 g
- Fiber 2 g
- Protein 3 g
- Cholesterol 17 mg
- Sugars 4 g
- Sodium 277 mg
- Potassium 384 mg

# Tomato, Kale White Beans Soup

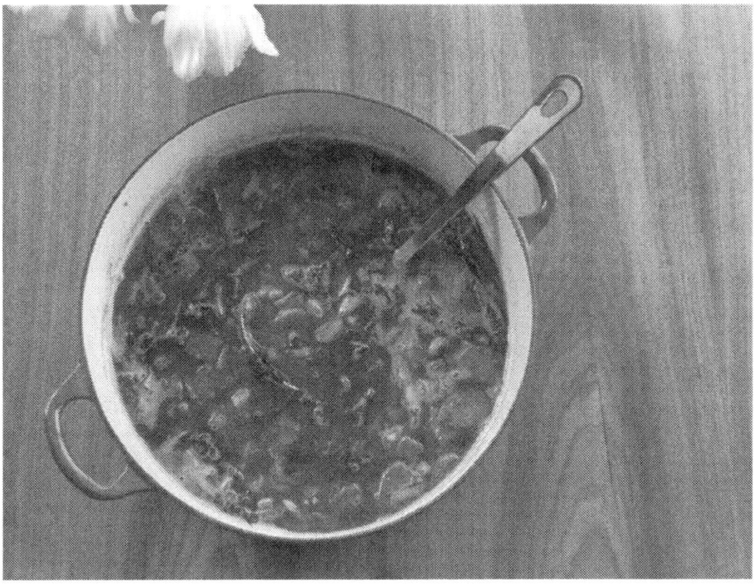

Up the ante of your tomato soup by adding kale and white beans. Make use of crushed or diced tomatoes for thicker texture.

**Serving size:** 4

**Preparation Cooking Time:** 10 minutes

**Ingredients:**

- 1 tablespoon olive oil
- 3 cups kale, chopped
- 1 teaspoon garlic, crushed and minced
- 28 oz. canned reduced-sodium tomato soup
- 14 oz. white beans (unsalted), rinsed and drained
- ¼ cup Parmesan cheese, grated

**Instructions:**

1. Pour the oil into a pan over medium heat.

2. Cook the kale and garlic for 30 seconds.

3. Pour the tomato soup into a pot.

4. Add the kale and beans to the pot.

5. Simmer for 3 minutes.

6. Top with the grated Parmesan cheese before serving.

**Nutrients per Serving:**

- Calories 200
- Fat 6 g
- Saturated fat 1 g
- Carbohydrates 29 g
- Fiber 6 g
- Protein 9 g
- Cholesterol 4 mg
- Sugars 1 g
- Sodium 355 mg
- Potassium 257 mg

# Mushroom Onion Soup

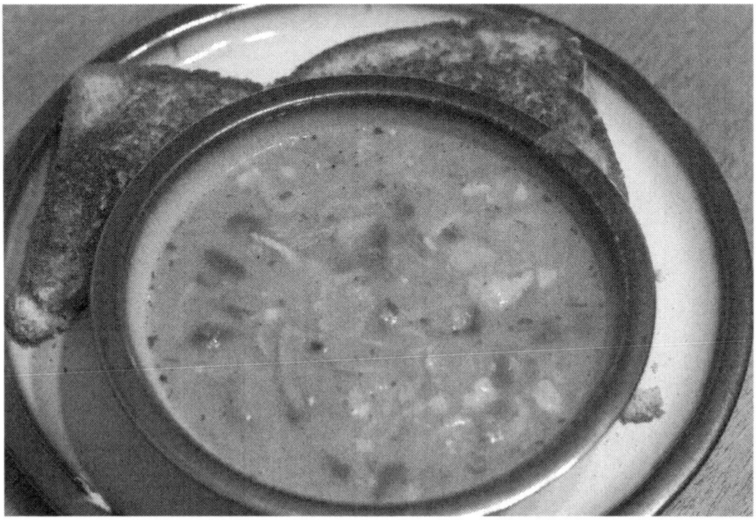

Spruce up your onion soup by adding mushroom slices and wild rice into the mix. This is a simple and hassle-free soup recipe that takes less than an hour to prepare.

**Serving size:** 4

**Preparation Cooking Time:** 40 minutes

**Ingredients:**

- 1 tablespoon olive oil
- 4 cups onion, sliced into cubes
- 1 cup leeks, sliced
- 2 teaspoons brown sugar
- 3 cups fresh mushrooms, sliced
- 2 carrots, chopped
- 14 oz. low-sodium chicken broth
- 2 cups water
- 1 ½ cups wild rice, cooked
- Pepper to taste
- ½ cup of cold water mixed with 2 tablespoons all-purpose flour

**Instructions:**

1. Pour the olive oil into a pan over medium heat.

2. Cook the onion and leeks in a pan over medium low heat for 15 minutes.

3. Stir in the sugar.

4. Cook for 5 minutes.

5. Add the carrots and mushrooms.

6. Cook for 3 minutes.

7. Pour in the broth, rice, pepper and water.

8. Cook for 1 minute.

9. Stir in the flour and water mixture.

10. Remove from heat and serve.

**Nutrients per Serving:**

- Calories 182
- Fat 3 g
- Saturated fat 0 g
- Carbohydrates 37 g
- Fiber 5 g
- Protein 5 g
- Cholesterol 0 mg
- Sugars 8 g
- Sodium 211 mg
- Potassium 431 mg

# Beef Veggie Soup

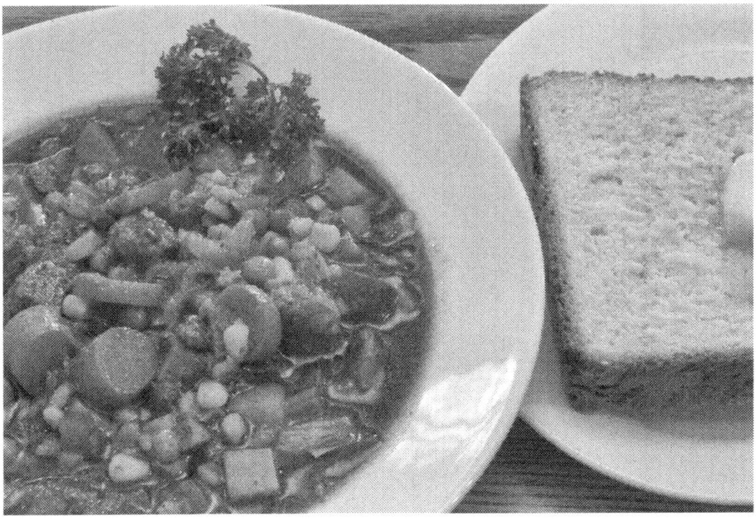

You only need 30 minutes active preparation to make this comforting beef and vegetable soup. It's the perfect antidote to a chilly winter night.

**Serving size:** 4

**Preparation Cooking Time:** 4 hours and 30 minutes

**Ingredients:**

- 1 lb. beef chuck roast, sliced into cubes
- 1 tablespoon vegetable oil
- 30 oz. canned diced tomatoes
- 1 cup water
- 2 potatoes, sliced into cubes
- 3 carrots, sliced into cubes
- 1 cup onion, chopped
- Salt to taste
- ½ teaspoon dried thyme
- ½ cup peas
- Parsley, chopped

**Instructions:**

1. In a pan over medium heat, pour the oil and cook the beef until brown.

2. Transfer the beef to a slow cooker.

3. Stir in the rest of the ingredients except the peas and parsley.

4. Cook on high for 4 hours.

5. Add the peas and garnish with the parsley before serving.

**Nutrients per Serving:**

- Calories 314
- Fat 8 g
- Saturated fat 2 g
- Carbohydrates 30 g
- Fiber 7 g
- Protein 30 g
- Cholesterol 50 mg
- Sugars 12 g
- Sodium 517 mg
- Potassium 847 mg

# Classic Tomato Soup

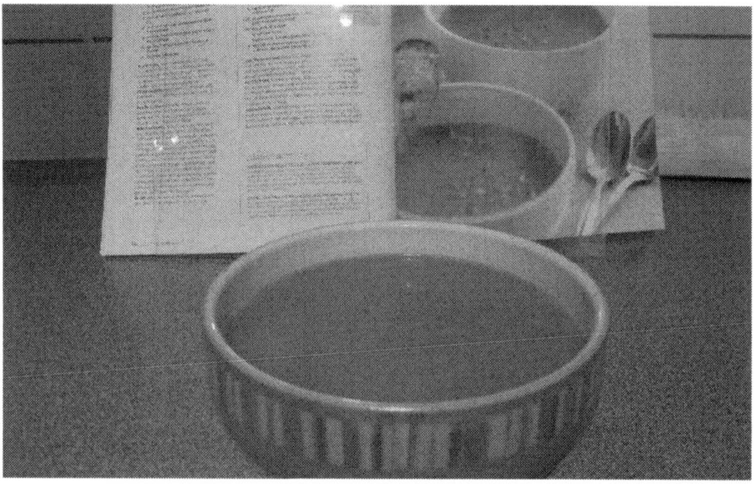

This is your favorite tomato soup that makes you remember your childhood years! It is made more special with the grilled cheese croutons.

**Serving size:** 6

**Preparation Cooking Time:** 30 minutes

**Ingredients:**

- 2 lb. tomatoes
- ¼ cup sweet onion, chopped
- ¼ cup fresh basil, chopped
- 1 cup sweet red peppers, chopped
- 1 cup vegetable broth (unsalted)
- 1 tablespoon honey
- 2 tablespoons heavy cream
- 4 grilled cheese croutons

**Instructions:**

1. Process the tomatoes, onions, basil, peppers and broth in a blender.

2. Blend until smooth.

3. Transfer to a saucepan.

4. Cook for 5 minutes.

5. Stir in the honey and cream.

6. Top with the cheese croutons.

**Nutrients per Serving:**

- Calories 69
- Fat 2 g
- Saturated fat 1 g
- Carbohydrates 11 g
- Fiber 2 g
- Protein 2 g
- Cholesterol 7 mg
- Sugars 8 g
- Sodium 105 mg
- Potassium 399 mg

# Carrot Parmesan Crackers

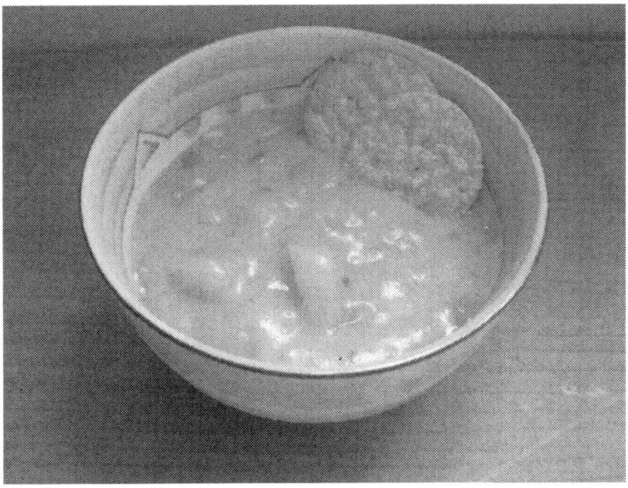

Snacking is truly a hard habit to break. But thankfully, you don't have to worry about ruining your diet when you make healthy and light snacks such as these crackers made with Parmesan cheese and shredded carrots.

**Serving size:** 18

**Preparation Cooking Time:** 1 hour

**Ingredients:**

- 1½ cups pastry flour
- 1 teaspoon baking powder
- ¼ teaspoon salt
- ¾ cup carrot, shredded
- 1 cup Parmesan cheese
- 2 teaspoons dried thyme, crushed
- ⅓ cup chilled butter, sliced into cubes
- ¼ cup water

**Instructions:**

1. Preheat your oven to 325 degrees F.

2. Mix the flour, baking powder, salt, carrot, Parmesan cheese and thyme in a bowl.

3. Fold in the butter and gradually add water.

4. Combine until consistency is crumbly.

5. Flatten into a square using a rolling pin.

6. Slice into rectangles.

7. Put these on your baking pan.

8. Bake for your 40 minutes. Let cool.

9. Store in airtight container.

**Nutrients per Serving:**

- Calories 109
- Fat 5 g
- Saturated fat 3 g
- Carbohydrates 13 g
- Fiber 2 g
- Protein 3 g
- Cholesterol 12 mg
- Sugars 0 g
- Sodium 139 mg
- Potassium 558 mg

# Stuffed Mushrooms

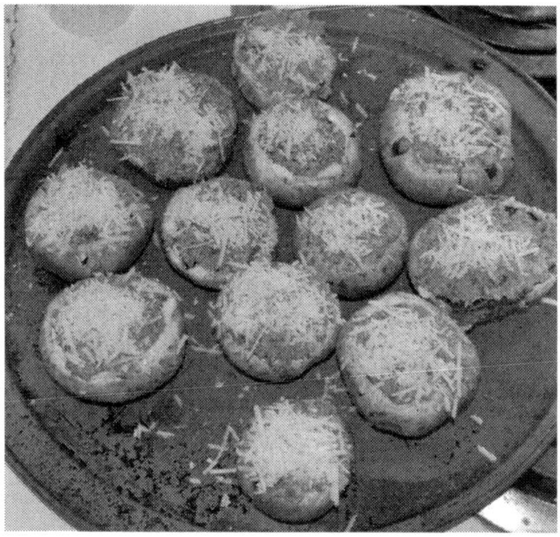

These mushroom caps stuffed with veggies and sour cream, topped with chopped broccoli will certainly be a hit in any get together.

**Serving size:** 12

**Preparation Cooking Time:** 25 minutes

**Ingredients:**

- 24 large mushrooms caps
- Cooking spray
- ¾ cup sour cream
- 1 green onion, minced
- 1 clove garlic, crushed and minced
- ½ cup sweet red pepper, chopped
- ½ cup carrot, chopped
- Salt and pepper to taste
- ¼ cup broccoli, chopped

**Instructions:**

1. Preheat your oven to 425 degrees F.

2. Line your baking sheet with foil.

3. Spray the mushrooms caps with oil.

4. Bake for 5 minutes.

5. In a bowl, combine the rest of the ingredients except the broccoli.

6. Stuff each of the mushroom caps with this mixture.

7. Top with the chopped broccoli.

**Nutrients per Serving:**

- Calories 29
- Fat 1 g
- Saturated fat 1 g
- Carbohydrates 3 g
- Fiber 0 g
- Protein 2 g
- Cholesterol 4 mg
- Sugars 0 g
- Sodium 26 mg
- Potassium 178 mg

# Cheesy Tomato Bites

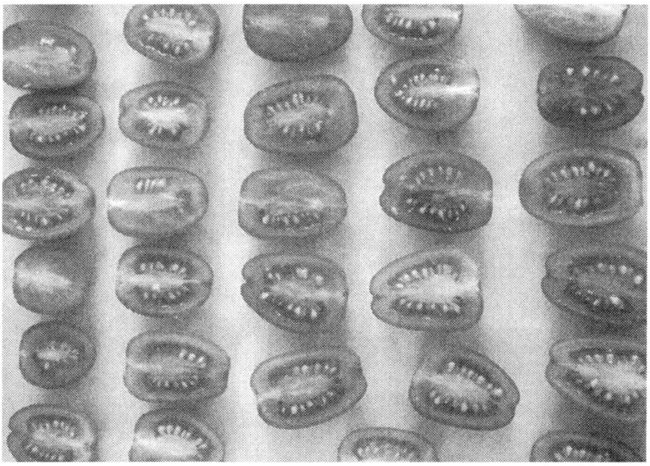

This is a simple appetizer that should definitely be part of your party menu. It's very easy to make and all your friends would love these cute little tomatoes.

**Serving size:** 6

**Preparation Cooking Time:** 15 minutes

**Ingredients:**

- 4 oz. mozzarella cheese, sliced into cubes
- 1 tablespoon white balsamic vinegar
- 2 tablespoons basil, chopped
- Pepper to taste
- 12 cherry tomatoes, sliced in half

**Instructions:**

1. Combine the mozzarella cubes, vinegar, pepper and basil.

2. Stuff the cherry tomatoes with mozzarella mixture.

**Nutrients per Serving:**

- Calories 106
- Fat 6 g
- Saturated fat 3 g
- Carbohydrates 6 g
- Fiber 1 g
- Protein 8 g
- Cholesterol 15 mg
- Sugars 4 g
- Sodium 188 mg
- Potassium 194 mg

# Sweet Potato Fries

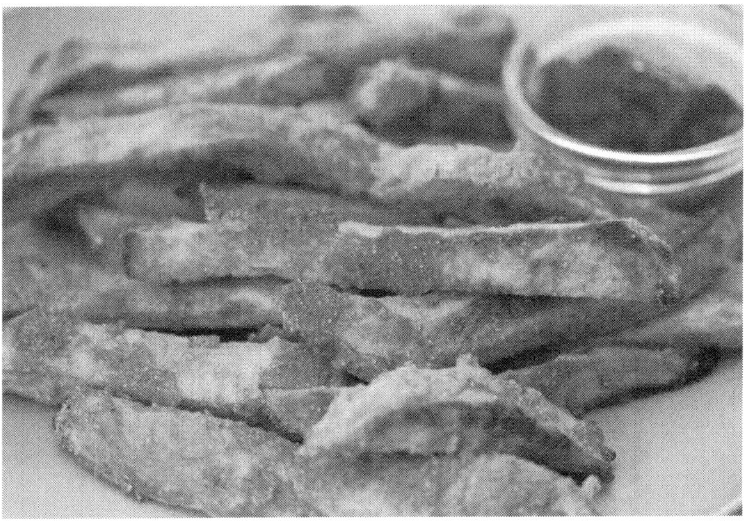

Craving for French fries but don't want the extra grease? Try this recipe—sweet potato fries. It's a quick and healthy snack that will surely satisfying your cravings.

**Serving size:** 4

**Preparation Cooking Time:** 30 minutes

**Ingredients:**

- 2 sweet potatoes, sliced into sticks
- 1 tablespoon olive oil
- ¼ teaspoon ground cinnamon
- ¼ teaspoon cayenne pepper
- Salt and pepper to taste

**Instructions:**

1. Preheat your oven to 350 degrees F.

2. Toss the sweet potatoes in olive oil.

3. Season with the cinnamon, cayenne, salt and pepper.

4. Bake in the oven until golden and crispy.

5. Let cool before serving.

**Nutrients per Serving:**

- Calories 84
- Fat 4 g
- Saturated fat 1 g
- Carbohydrates 12 g
- Fiber 2 g
- Protein 1 g
- Cholesterol 0 mg
- Sugars 4 g
- Sodium 166 mg
- Potassium 276 mg

# Garlic Mashed Potatoes

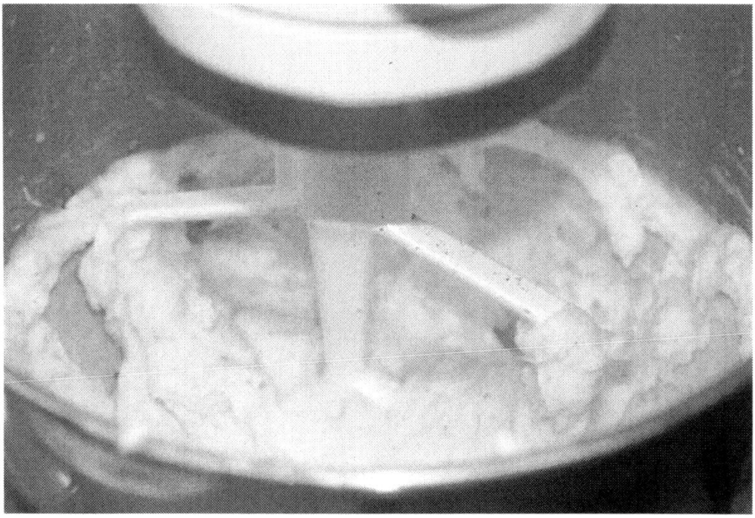

Mashed potatoes are so popular as a side dish, you can pair it up with almost any main course, whether it's grilled beef, fried chicken, steak and many more. This one is a step up from the usual mashed potatoes as garlic lends it extra flavor, and buttermilk makes it extra creamy.

**Serving size:** 6

**Preparation Cooking Time:** 50 minutes

**Ingredients:**

- 4 cups water
- 1½ lb. potatoes, sliced into cubes
- 5 cloves garlic, roasted and mashed into paste
- ½ cup buttermilk
- 4 tablespoons butter
- Salt to taste

**Instructions:**

1. Pour the water into a pot.

2. Add steamer basket inside.

3. Put the potatoes on top of the steamer.

4. Steam for 40 minutes.

5. Mash the potatoes with a fork.

6. Stir in the garlic, milk, butter and salt.

**Nutrients per Serving:**

- Calories 174
- Fat 8 g
- Saturated fat 5 g
- Carbohydrates 24 g
- Fiber 2 g
- Protein 3 g
- Cholesterol 21 mg
- Sugars 2 g
- Sodium 240 mg
- Potassium 400 mg

# Fruit Parfait with Yogurt

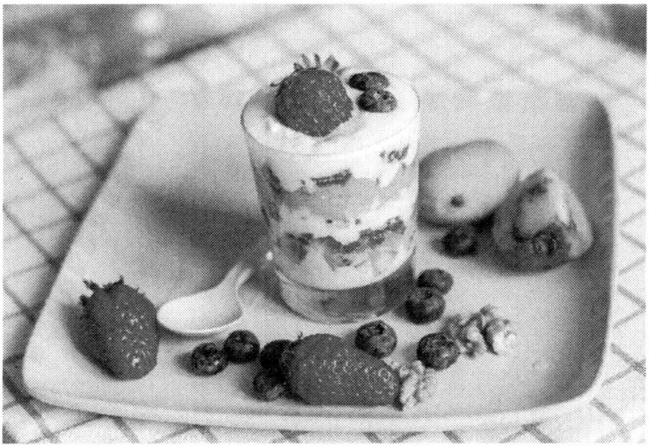

A quick and healthy dessert that will cap a wonderful meal—this fruit parfait with yogurt comes together within only a few minutes.

**Serving size:** 4

**Preparation Cooking Time:** 15 minutes

**Ingredients:**

- ½ low-fat cream cheese
- 16 oz. plain yogurt
- 1½ cups strawberries, sliced
- 1½ cups peaches, chopped
- 1 cup blueberries, sliced
- 2 tablespoons walnuts, toasted

**Instructions:**

1. Beat all the cream cheese using an electric mixer for 30 seconds.

2. Add the yogurt and mix for another 30 seconds.

3. Toss the fruits in a bowl.

4. Layer the fruit and yogurt mixture in a glass jar.

5. Sprinkle the walnuts on top.

6. Chill in the refrigerator before serving.

**Nutrients per Serving:**

- Calories 206
- Fat 9 g
- Saturated fat 4 g
- Carbohydrates 25 g
- Fiber 4 g
- Protein 8 g
- Cholesterol 23 mg
- Sugars 4 g
- Sodium 163 mg
- Potassium 559 mg

# Oatmeal Muffins with Rhubarb

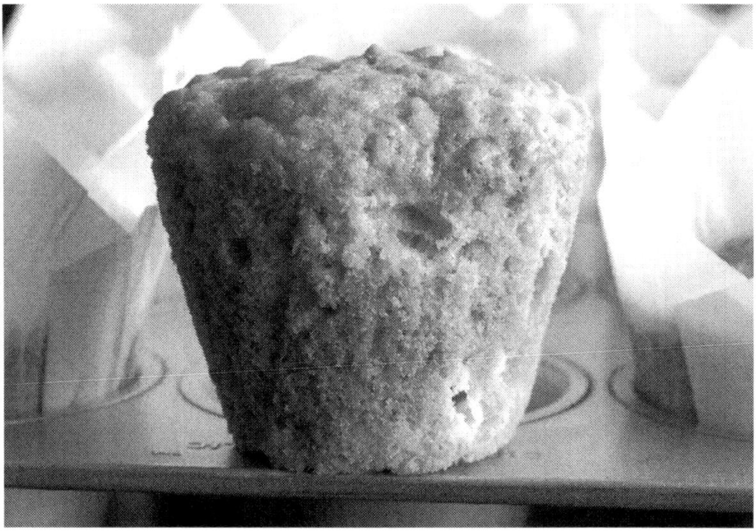

These oatmeal muffins taste as great as they look! These have just the right amount of sweetness and packs in a lot of crunch that you'd surely enjoy with every bite.

**Serving size:** 12

**Preparation Cooking Time:** 45 minutes

**Ingredients:**

- Cooking spray

**Muffins:**

- 2 cups rolled oats, divided
- ½ cup all-purpose flour
- 1 cup whole wheat flour
- ½ cup brown sugar
- ¼ teaspoon salt
- ¾ cup buttermilk
- 2 eggs, beaten
- 1 teaspoon baking powder
- 2 tablespoons vegetable oil
- 1 teaspoon vanilla
- ½ teaspoon baking soda
- 1 cup rhubarb, chopped

**Topping:**

- ½ teaspoon ground cinnamon
- ¼ cup walnuts, chopped

**Instructions:**

1. Preheat your oven to 350 degrees F.

2. Line your muffin pan with baking cups.

3. Spray each one with oil.

4. Put the rolled oats in a food processor.

5. Pulse until finely ground.

6. Put the ground oats in a bowl.

7. Stir in the flours, baking powder, baking soda, sugar and salt.

8. Mix well.

9. Create a well in the middle part of the bowl.

10. Put the rest of the muffin ingredients in center and mix well.

11. Mix with the rest of the flour mixture.

12. Add the mixture to the muffin cups.

13. Top with the cinnamon and walnuts.

14. Bake for 20 to 25 minutes.

**Nutrients per Serving:**

- Calories 181
- Fat 5 g
- Carbohydrates 30 g
- Protein 5 g
- Fiber 3 g
- Saturated fat 1 g
- Cholesterol 1 mg
- Sugars 11 g
- Sodium 180 mg
- Potassium 76 mg

# Strawberry on Graham Crackers

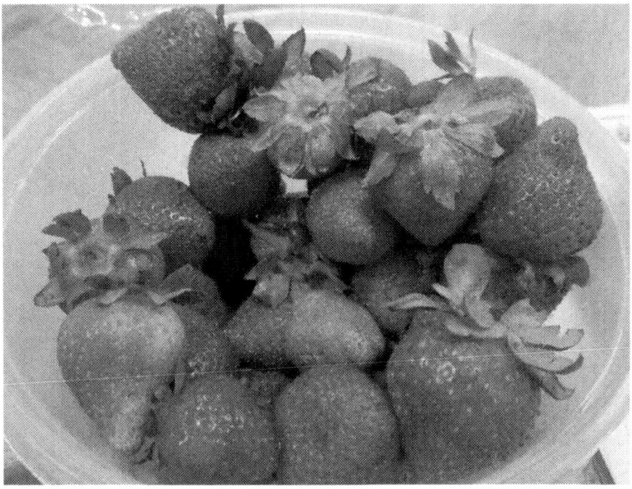

This is an attractive and delicious dessert recipe that will only take you 5 minutes or less to whip up. Caution though: these bites are most likely gone in 30 seconds!

**Serving size:** 4

**Preparation Cooking Time:** 5 minutes

**Ingredients:**

- 8 graham crackers
- 8 teaspoons cream cheese
- 8 strawberries, sliced

**Instructions:**

1. Divide the graham crackers to make rectangles.

2. Spread the cream cheese on top of each rectangle.

3. Add the strawberry slices on top.

**Nutrients per Serving:**

- Calories 90
- Fat 3 g
- Saturated fat 1 g
- Carbohydrates 13 g
- Fiber 1 g
- Protein 2 g
- Cholesterol 7 mg
- Sugars 6 g
- Sodium 114 mg
- Potassium 56 mg

# Banana Choco Chip Muffins

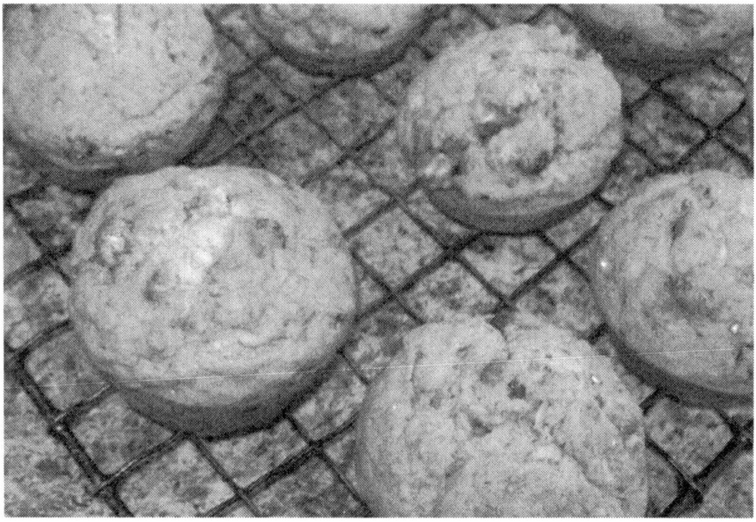

Choco chips cookies and banana muffins rolled into one in this hassle-free dessert that you can store and enjoy for up to a week.

**Serving size:** 24

**Preparation Cooking Time:** 50 minutes

**Ingredients:**

- Cooking spray
- 1½ cups rolled oats
- ¼ teaspoon baking soda
- 1 teaspoon baking powder
- ¼ teaspoon salt
- 2 eggs
- 2 ripe bananas, mashed
- ¼ cup brown sugar
- 3 tablespoons vegetable oil
- 1 teaspoon vanilla extract
- ½ cup mini chocolate chips

**Instructions:**

1. Preheat your oven to 350 degrees F.

2. Spray your muffin pan with oil.

3. Put the oats in a food processor.

4. Process until finely ground.

5. Stir in the baking soda, salt and baking powder.

6. Add the rest of the ingredients except the chocolate chips.

7. Pulse for a few seconds.

8. Pour the mixture into the muffin pan.

9. Top with the chocolate chips.

10. Bake for 15 minutes.

**Nutrients per Serving:**

- Calories 78
- Fat 4 g
- Saturated fat 1 g
- Carbohydrates 11 g
- Fiber 1 g
- Protein 1 g
- Cholesterol 16 mg
- Sugars 6 g
- Sodium 65 mg
- Potassium 77 mg

# Oatmeal Cookies with Dried Fruits

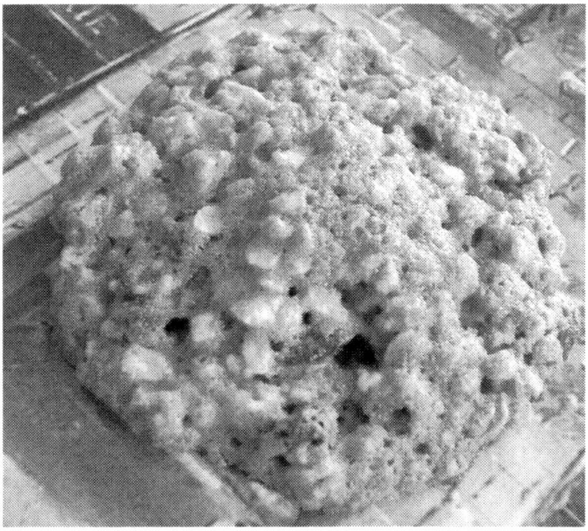

Step up the game by adding dried fruits to your oatmeal cookies. Not only does this mean more flavor, this also increases the cookie's nutritional content.

**Serving size:** 48

**Preparation Cooking Time:** 35 minutes

**Ingredients:**

- 2 cups rolled oats
- Cooking spray
- ½ cup butter, softened
- ¾ teaspoon baking soda
- ¼ teaspoon ground allspice
- ¼ teaspoon salt
- 1½ cups brown sugar
- 2 eggs, beaten
- 1 teaspoon vanilla
- 6 oz. yogurt
- 2¼ cups flour
- ¼ cup dried apricots, sliced
- ¼ cup dried currants
- ¼ cup walnuts, toasted and chopped

**Instructions:**

1. Preheat your oven to 375 degrees F.
2. Spread the oats on a baking pan.
3. Bake for 10 minutes.
4. Spray your cookie pan with oil.
5. Beat all the butter using an electric mixer for 30 seconds.
6. Stir in the baking soda, allspice, salt and sugar.
7. Beat until well mixed.
8. Add the egg, vanilla and yogurt.
9. Stir in the flour, dried fruits and walnuts.
10. Create cookies from the mixture.
11. Bake for 10 to 12 minutes or until golden brown.
12. Let cool before serving.

**Nutrients per Serving:**

- Calories 101
- Fat 3 g
- Saturated fat 1 g
- Carbohydrates 17 g
- Fiber 1 g
- Protein 2 g
- Cholesterol 5 mg
- Sugars 8 g
- Sodium 55 mg
- Potassium 73 mg

# Conclusion

For sure, you're excited to try all these delicious recipes.

Now that you're aware how excessive sodium can affect your health; you can take a step towards a healthier diet.

Along with lowering sodium intake, it would also be a good idea to also reduce consumption of sugar, fats, and cholesterol.

Maintaining a healthy and well-balanced diet can do wonders not only for your physical health but for the overall quality of your life.

# About the Author

A native of Albuquerque, New Mexico, Sophia Freeman found her calling in the culinary arts when she enrolled at the Sante Fe School of Cooking. Freeman decided to take a year after graduation and travel around Europe, sampling the cuisine from small bistros and family owned restaurants from Italy to Portugal. Her bubbly personality and inquisitive nature made her popular with the locals in the villages and when she finished her trip and came home, she had made friends for life in the places she had visited. She also came home with a deeper understanding of European cuisine.

Freeman went to work at one of Albuquerque's 5-star restaurants as a sous-chef and soon worked her way up to head chef. The restaurant began to feature Freeman's original dishes as specials on the menu and soon after, she began to write e-books with her recipes. Sophia's dishes mix local flavours with European inspiration making them irresistible to the diners in her restaurant and the online community.

Freeman's experience in Europe didn't just teach her new ways of cooking, but also unique methods of presentation. Using rich sauces, crisp vegetables and meat cooked to perfection, she creates a stunning display as well as a delectable dish. She has won many local awards for her cuisine and she continues to delight her diners with her culinary masterpieces.

# Author's Afterthoughts

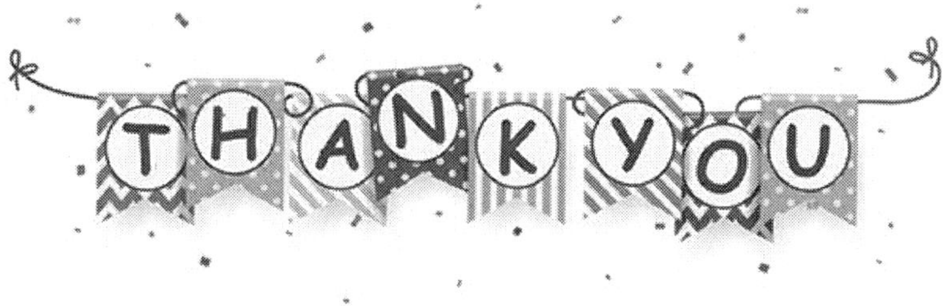


I want to convey my big thanks to all of my readers who have taken the time to read my book. Readers like you make my work so rewarding and I cherish each and every one of you.

Grateful cannot describe how I feel when I know that someone has chosen my work over all of the choices available online. I hope you enjoyed the book as much as I enjoyed writing it.

Feedback from my readers is how I grow and learn as a chef and an author. Please take the time to let me know your thoughts by leaving a review on Amazon so I and your fellow readers can learn from your experience.

***My deepest thanks,***

***Sophia Freeman***

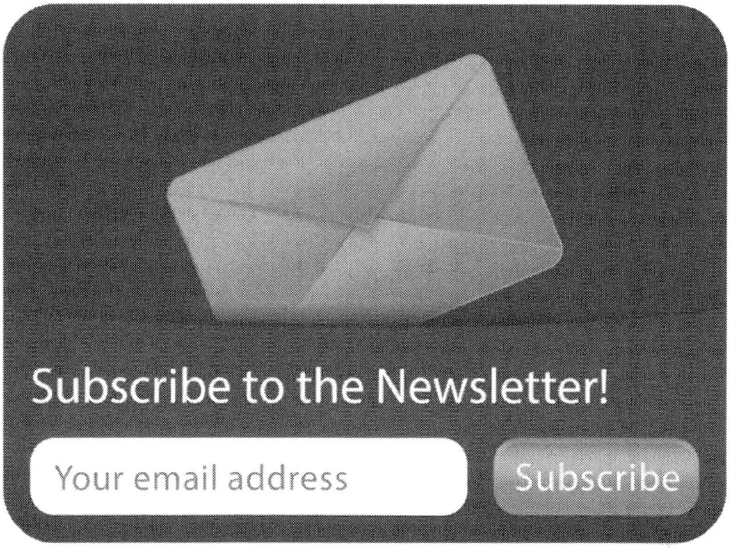


https://sophia.subscribemenow.com/

Printed in Great Britain
by Amazon

33454832R00104